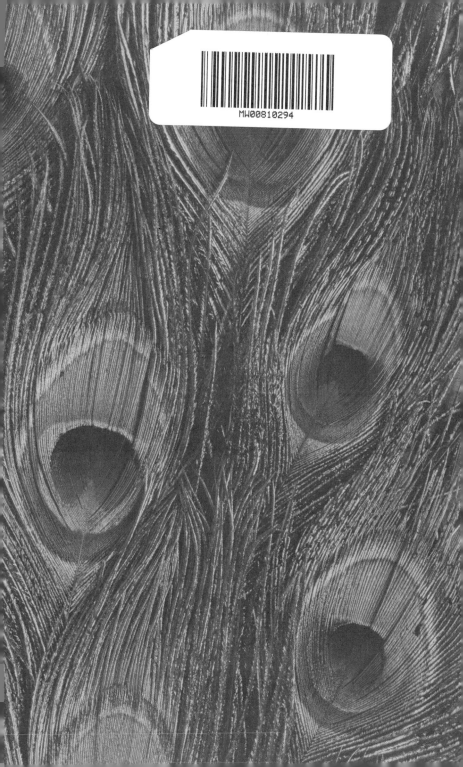

MW00810294

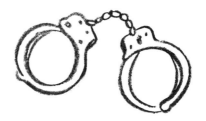

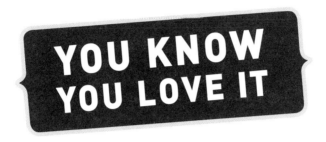

Lessons in
Sexual Mischief

dominatrix **ILONA PARIS**, M.Ed.

Illustrations by woolypear

Stewart Tabori & Chang
NEW YORK

Published in 2008 by Stewart, Tabori & Chang
An imprint of Harry N. Abrams, Inc.

Library of Congress Cataloging-in-Publication Data
Paris, Ilona.
You know you love it : lessons in sexual mischief / Ilona Paris.
p. cm.
ISBN 978-1-58479-626-8
1. Sexual dominance and submission. 2. Sex instruction. I. Title.
HQ79.P26 2007
306.77'5—dc22   2007022867

Editor: Ann Treistman
Designer: woolypear
Production Manager: Jacqueline Poirier

Printed and bound in the U.S.A.
10 9 8 7 6 5 4 3 2 1

HNA ■■■■■
harry n. abrams, inc.

115 West 18th Street
New York, NY 10011
www.hnabooks.com

Disclaimer: The following is not indicative of the full extent of S&M practices that
I used as a professional dominatrix. While the focus is on heterosexuality, I warmly
welcome readers of all erotic minorities who practice alternative lifestyles.

Dedicated to my Aunt Claire and Uncle Ray who told me I better get it together before the rapture. <eyes rolling>

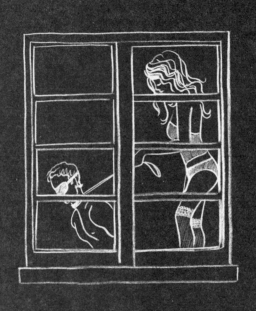

"Desire begins with taboo."

—Gore Vidal

contents

10 SEXUAL MISCHIEF: AN INTRO

22 DISCOVERING MY KINK

38 A LEOPARD IS BORN

54 IT'S ALL IN HOW YOU SAY IT

72 CAKEALICIOUS

88 OF HUMAN BONDAGE

106 FOR THE SPANKER IN YOU

122 WHIP IT GOOD

138 THE FEMININE FACTOR

154 YOU MAY KISS MY FEET

172 BUTTING IN

188 VACATION SEX

208 DUNGEON SALE

218 THE NITTY GRITTY

237 *The Paris Report* Methodology

238 Bibliography

240 Acknowledgments

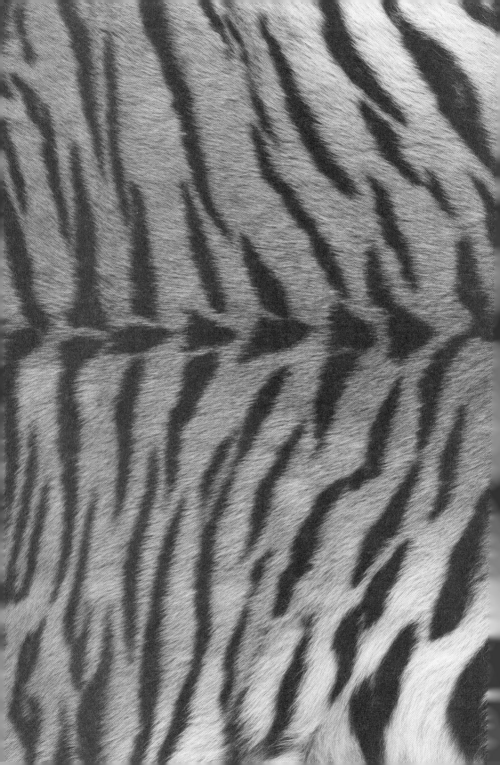

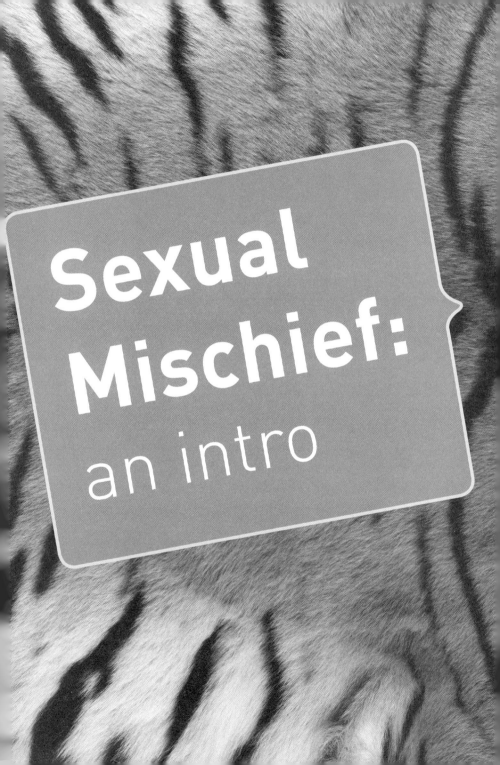

Sexual Mischief:
an intro

"We must realize that we are evolution."
—Teilhard de Chardin

Ask most people what they think when they hear S&M, and most likely they'd say this:

"Ew, scary!"

Or this:

"Ow!"

Or even this:

"Sick!"

How wrong they'd be.

How much they'd be missing out on.

In truth, S&M is one of the most playful, fun, mischievous, and good-humored practices you can engage in. Those loaded initials pack a wallop of teasing, lighthearted sexuality that can do much for so many, from setting a young woman apart from her competitors in the sexual arena of the modern meat market, to spicing up a love life for long-married couples who're bored with the same old same old.

And not only that, but chances are that some variation of S&M is already a part of your life, whether you know it or not.

If you've ever playfully bitten a partner during intercourse . . .

Or stroked an inner thigh with a feather . . .

Or nibbled whipped cream off a nipple . . .

Or run an ice cube across the flat of a back . . .

You were engaging in what I call "Sexual Mischief."

Not the hard-core whips-and-chains variety, maybe—though that can be delicious, too. (Wait till you see!) But right now we're talking about the softer, sexual mischief side, Ilona's brand of S&M.

It doesn't even have to be overtly sexual. If you've ever received a friendly pinch on the butt that kind of made you tingle, deep inside . . .

Or had a friend scratch a hard-to-reach itch on your back . . . a little harder . . . a little harder . . . a scratch so hard it hurt . . .

Or given a lover a playful smack on the butt cheek . . .

Just because it felt so damn good . . .

A good that went straight to the groin . . .

Then you, too, were engaging in Sexual Mischief (definition follows).

Here's the thing that most people don't understand: Far from being decadent or nasty (well, it can be those things, too, but we'll get to that later), at its heart S&M is all about innocence. The innocence of childhood play. The innocence of frolicking on a new-mown lawn, enjoying the sensations of being alive with all your nimble limbs and your bright nerve-endings and your devious little imagination, which is the most entertaining part of all.

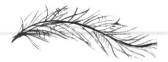

ILONA'S DEFINITIONS

Let's define our terms, shall we? The world has a lot of ways of abbreviating the erotic arts, but here's how we'll do it:

S&M or S/M

The abbreviation for sadomasochism, pure and simple—the receiving or giving of pain for pleasure and sexual gratification.

B/D

The abbreviation for bondage and domination. Bondage allows the submissive to release him or herself to the power of another individual. Domination is for people who find it stimulating to be in control of another individual.

D/S

Dominance and submission, in which the dynamics of power and control are used to sexually enhance a relationship.

BDSM

The umbrella term for bondage, domination, sadism, and masochism.

THE SCENE

A community of people involved in BSDM.

Sexual Mischief

Ilona's brand of sexual mischief, otherwise known as "kink." This may include elements from all of the above—from softer than soft to harder than hard, in which you let your imagination run riot. No rules, no boundaries, sheer erotic fun but always safe, sane, and consensual.

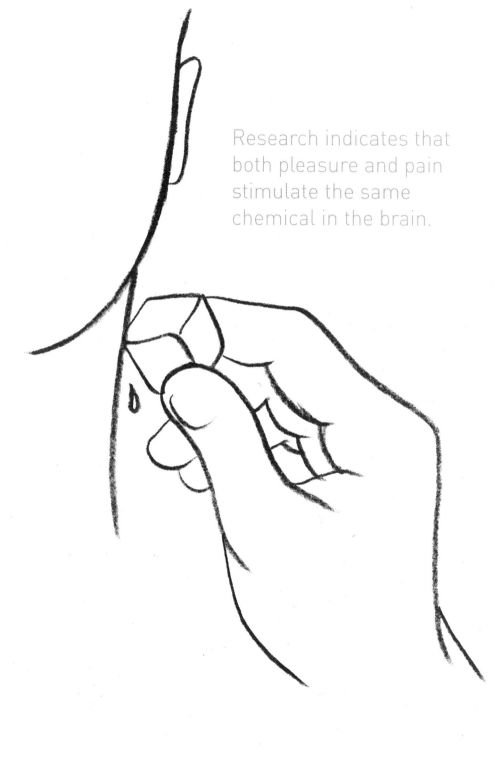

Research indicates that both pleasure and pain stimulate the same chemical in the brain.

The little-known truth is that just about all of us played S&M games when we were small, before stodgy old self-consciousness set in and ruined our fun.

If you've ever wrestled a cousin on the carpet in the TV room (when *The Brady Bunch* got boring) . . .

Or pinned your little brother to the driveway and wouldn't let him up till he cried, "Uncle" . . .

Or let yourself be tied up by a best friend and tickled till tears ran down your cheeks . . .

Or dared someone to tell you a secret hankering they'd never told anyone before . . .

Then you've been there, baby.

Welcome back.

And here's the funny thing about being an adult, tapping back into this kind of childish innocence.

It gives you power like you've never had in your life.

"For over a century, people who engaged in bondage, beatings and humiliation for sexual pleasure were considered mentally ill. . . . What's new is that such desires are increasingly being considered normal, even healthy, as experts begin to recognize their potential psychological value."

— *Marianne Apostolides*, Psychology Today

WAS EDMUND BURKE A PAIN FREAK?

The eighteenth-century Anglo-Irish statesman and philosopher Edmund Burke defined the sensation of pleasure derived from pain with one word: "sublime." He was on to something.

Imagine this scenario:

You've just had a good caning. Your ass stings so good. You're still giggling inside from all the dark little mischief you incurred, and all the playful goodness you were able to spark with another human being.

Then you go to the office. You get up to lead a meeting at the boardroom, and beneath that Prada suit, your ass is still burning! You're suffused with the knowledge of what you are secretly capable of.

What you allowed yourself to explore.

What you gave yourself permission to feel.

The dimension of sexuality that you dared to bring to the light of day.

How daring.

How devilish.

How freeing.

How . . . empowering.

Because if you can do that, you . . . can . . . do . . . anything.

I should know. I've earned my psychology degrees by studying all the technical tomes about what turns people on and why. Then, to continue my education, I became a member of the Scene myself—a genuine red-blooded dominatrix who knows how to wield a whip and light a man on fire. Literally.

If you're reading this book, I'd guess that you have some devious little part of yourself that suspects there might be more to sex than what you've experienced thus far in life. Maybe you want to try some bondage, or even whipping. Would it be so very wrong to get a little pleasure from pain, whether you are inflicting or receiving it? (Might the wrongness itself be part of the thrill?) Or from the way you leave your everyday life behind during those moments of anticipation and ecstasy? Wherever you are in your erotic journey through life—whether you're on a second date and want to make an indelible impression, or you've been married thirty years and want to bring some heat back to the bedroom, or you're already in the Scene and need some fresh ideas—I'm going to give you the edge by taking elements from my experience in both my dungeon and my office.

PARADOXICAL PAIN

On the most basic level, BDSM in all of its permutations involves a limited amount of physical pain. Pain is paradoxical: Yes, it hurts, but when strictly controlled, it also allows for the release of endorphins—that mysterious group of opiate-like peptides which spark a sensation akin to a runner's high or the afterglow of orgasm. Submissives relish this feeling so much they call it "subspace."

Here's the deal. You don't have to have had an abused childhood, or be a twisted adult, to be attracted to S&M. Millions of normal, well-adjusted people practice some aspect of it— and reap its benefits—in the privacy of their everyday suburban homes. When I was a pro Domme (professional dominatrix), my typical client was a responsible father of two, a computer geek or doctor with a gourmet kitchen and a $600,000 mortgage. I've seen professors, professional basketball players, and well-known radio personalities in my dungeon.

It isn't, in other words, the outer fringe any longer. It's as close as your neighbor's playroom . . . after the kiddies are put to bed.

"Sadomasochism is embedded in our culture since our culture operates on the basis of dominant and submissive relationships, and aggression is socially valued." — *John K. Noyes*

Let's face it: kinky sex is far more fun than vanilla pudding. It's more like eating chocolate while the creamy inside squirts in your mouth and down your fingers. It's also incredibly empowering. For the person in control, it's a safe opportunity to act out the thrill of having complete sovereignty over another human being. For the person being controlled, it's a chance to let go of all the responsibilities of life—a total surrender of the ego. For both, it's a healthy release, surprisingly similar to the release one gets from a successful therapy session—a pressure valve for busy people who need a little relief from the stresses of modern life.

And here's the kicker: You'll be amazed at what a little sexual mischief can do for the ordinary sex life. Believe me, it can be one of the greatest picker-uppers for bored, tired libidos. As I say in the pages to come, creative erotica is the salt and pepper of the sex world. Did you know, for instance, that men adore having a woman breathe warm air through the fabric of their crotches, with a

Pain is not the end-all of sexual mischief, but only one aspect of the sexual cosmos that also includes service, humiliation, anticipation, submission, and domination. S&M is not strictly about sensation.

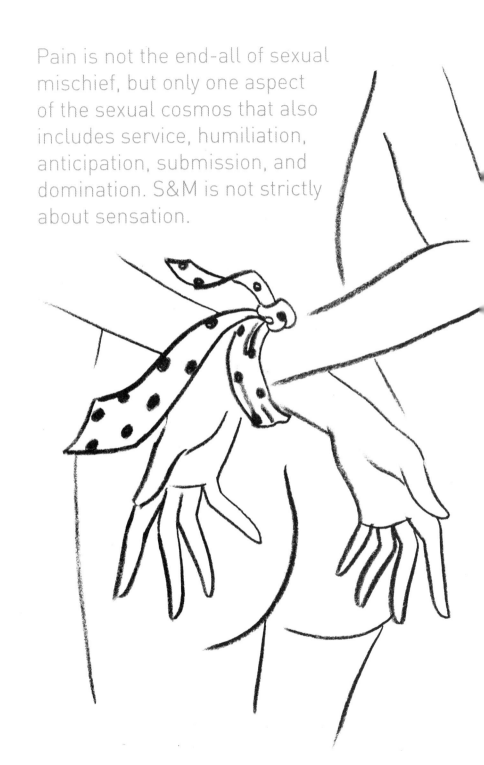

strategic nip thrown in for good measure? It's a little-known secret that men are far more into what I call "soft sensuals" than they let on. A man loves to be blindfolded from behind and have his partner surprise him with a dirty little whisper in his ear. Powerlessness is the ultimate turn-on for men, so they can just relax and think with their cocks.

And get this—it's one sexual technique that actually gets better with age. Most of the time it doesn't even become part of one's lifestyle until midlife. As a woman gets older and more refined, she can turn herself into the kind of sex goddess she only dreamed of being when she was twenty.

Y'know, there are a lot of sex books for and by women on the market lately. And that's all to the good. Call girl confessionals, teenage tell-alls, self-help guides, erotic novels, photographic treatments, and histories of sexual particulars are whetting everyone's appetite. A growing genre of extreme female confession— from nymphomaniac picaresques to spanking fetishes to the joy of anal sex—are literate ticklers to the mysteries of sadomasochism.

What goes on between a man and a woman in a domination session? Who exactly does the hurting, and how much? Why does the hurt feel so good? What sex secrets are known by Dommes that make well-known politicians and high-powered businessmen fall in love with them?

I'm excited to share with you—in intimate, luxuriant detail— how sexually thrilling it is to be a woman in command of her body, her power, and the full dimension of sadomasochism—the ultimate erotic art.

Curious? Your education is about to begin.

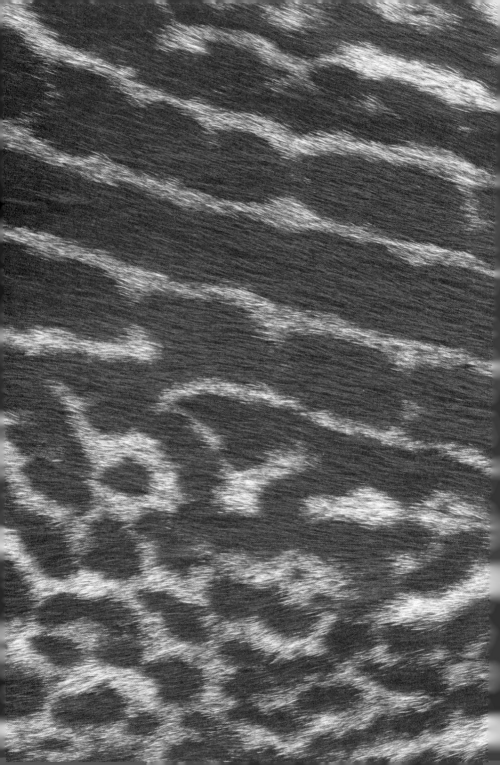

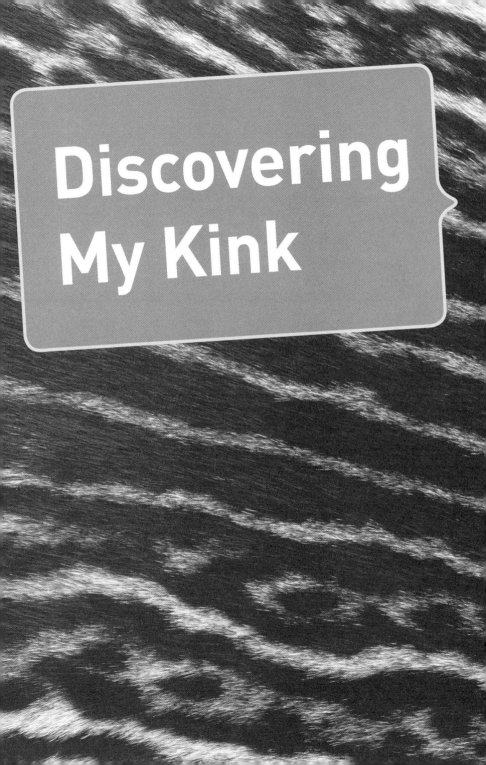

Discovering My Kink

*I wasn't born a pro Domme.
I had to grow into it.
I tried out many things first.*

I fell in love with *The Story of O* when I was nineteen. The book was about BDSM, particularly dominance and submission, and it went straight to my clit. In the last chapter, O is brought to the woods where she is told to lift her dress in front of her Master. She wears only garters and stockings. She is given a rose with thorns and told to place it between her stocking and her thigh. The piercing of her skin, the exposure of her pussy, the humiliation of presenting it openly to another human being still gets me wet when I think about it now.

In another scene, O is in a fine restaurant with her Master. She is told to stand when the waiter arrives. Her Master and another gentleman finger her cunt as the waiter asks her if there is anything he can get her. That moment of excitement, the pure titillation from the dominant/submissive interaction, hit a nerve within my being. It sat embedded in me for many years, patiently waiting to be released.

Over the early years of my sexual adventuring, I never delved into the realm of masochism or sadism. Once in a while there was a mild spanking or a little slap in the face—but never ultimate submission or the empowerment of dominance that I'd read about in *O*. The possibility of it didn't really enter my mind. I liked sex, knew I was passionate, and knew I was open to delving into the unusual. But the unusual never blossomed for me until my thirties, when I found myself reading more.

As everyone knows, reading can broaden one's horizons. I started reading the erotic adventures of *The Claiming of Sleeping Beauty* by A. N. Roquelaure (Anne Rice writing under a pseudonym), an adult fairy tale in which Beauty is the bound captive of an Eastern sultan and is kept prisoner in a castle. Rice makes what is considered the forbidden side of passion a doorway into the hidden regions of the psyche and the heart. Needless to say, I found it extremely arousing.

I was married at the time to a man I loved very much, but who was incapable of having down-and-dirty, steaming sex with me. It just wasn't in his nature. So I took matters into my own hands and went to a women's sex store in Coolidge Corner called Grand Orgasm. (Funny thing—Boston has a reputation for being straight-laced, a result of its Puritanical history, I guess, but in reality it's a beehive of sexual buzz. As in many cities around the globe, you can practically hear the *hummm* if you let your ears attune themselves to it.) A wonderful pervert named Kerry Airy ran the store. Bless her soul, she conducted terrific classes out of this little shop—classes on fisting, stripping for your lover, and Intro to S&M. Well, I liked the latter so much I took it twice. Oink, oink.

I went to the first class by myself. I was excited. I certainly had no idea what to expect, but was ready for anything. Kerry ran the class, and two other people participated in it with her. I later found out this was called a "scene." The scene took place in an office where two female employers punished a male employee for his misdemeanors. He was made to strip down to his underwear and was forced to lick the women's black high-heeled pumps. He then had to kneel on the floor while they took a leather riding crop and slapped his bare bottom with it.

I was onto something here. It was dangerous and exciting. It made me feel alive and challenged. The sheer audacity of it went directly to my CirClit City, as it were. Afterwards, members of the audience walked around the shop looking at the various sex toys on the shelves: black leather, chains, whips, and handcuffs. *Mmm*, yummy. I was standing in front of a row of vibrators when a luscious-looking woman, a high-powered attorney as it turned out, came up to me to discuss a particular fuchsia dildo. She was obviously trying to slap the make on me. I was scared as hell and couldn't follow her lead. But it was so exciting.

> Yes, even Ilona Paris gets nervous sometimes! No one is born hardwired to accept this much excitement, you know. Sometimes we just have to screw up our courage, as it were.

I wanted in on this Scene, whatever this Scene was. At that point I was vanilla, which means a person who is not a practitioner of alternative sexual lifestyles such as BDSM. Just learning the terminology sent shivers down my spine.

ILONA'S FAVORITE SEX BOOKS

Beauty's Punishment by A. N. Roquelaure

Beauty's Release by A. N. Roquelaure

The Claiming of Sleeping Beauty by A. N. Roquelaure

Delta of Venus by Anaïs Nin

Domina by Gloria Brame

Emmanuelle by Emmanuelle Arsan

The 43rd Mistress by Grant Andrews

The Happy Hooker by Xaviera Hollander

Parachutes and Kisses by Erica Jong

The Story of O by Pauline Reage

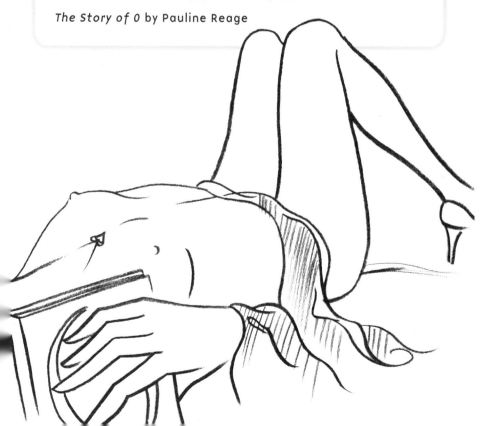

Between five and ten percent of people
have experimented with sadomasochism
(S&M), which is most popular among
educated, middle- and upper-middle-
class men and women, according to the
National Coalition for Sexual Freedom.

I hit the personals. Number three was a man who was to become my Dom. His name was Ivan. His profile on the Internet was compelling. It read:

Member Name:	*Sir*
Location:	*Boston, MA*
Sex:	*Male*
Marital Status:	*Single Dom*
Hobbies:	*Exploring psyches—pushing limits—empowering submissives—expanding intellects—demanding excellence. I seek those who are brave and passionate enough to embrace what makes them question, tremble & yearn, who are exceptionally intelligent and giving.*
	I have no patience for the timid. Keep repeating my name, and we will get along fine. :)
Occupation:	*Architect - builder - developer - dominant.*
Personal Quote:	*Commit to your passions.*

Our first meeting was fraught with electricity. I had to drive Shirley, my little yellow Beetle, to his house to meet him in Watertown because he didn't have a car. He had female submissives drive him everywhere. I found this out later. He gave me directions to his house. I got lost and was quite irate by the time I arrived at his impressively huge stucco house. (He never bothered to correct me by admitting that he was just renting the top floor.) I walked up the steps. The doors were open. No one was around at first. There were French antiques and nineteenth-century books all over the place.

THE PARIS REPORT

All of the things I'm telling you in this book are backed up by clinical research, both from my years as a licensed psychotherapist working with people in the Scene, and from the Paris Report, the survey I created and conducted with hundreds of members of this world. In the Paris Report, respondents answered such questions as what age people are when they start to have kinky thoughts, the education level of kinksters, and their history of sexual abuse. The Paris Report— envisioned as a kind of Kinsey Report of sadomasochism— not only provides valuable information about which people have been speculating for years, but will also help the clinician in supporting erotic minorities as well as letting laymen know they are not alone in their sexual preferences.

(See page 237 for more detail.)

And then I saw him. He was a big man, wearing khaki green shorts and a linen shirt with the sleeves rolled up. He was not wearing shoes, and his toenails looked like they'd never been cut. I thought I was going to be sick. He had a shock of white hair—I later learned that his friends called him Great White—with piercing brown eyes, and when he said "Hello" in a deep, resonating voice, I was drawn to him despite myself. We sat on his deck, with a railing around it that didn't look very sturdy. Now I was physically on edge, as well as psychologically. He sipped from a glass of chardonnay while I drank mango juice. I didn't know what to expect from this guy. I mean, was he going to order me to crawl on the floor right away, or chain me up and whip me? I could hardly sit still.

When you enter the world of S&M, and all its luxurious trappings, the anticipation of what is going to happen is a large part of the thrill. This evening was no different. I was ready to jump out of my skin because all I could think about was what this man was going to do. When would something happen, and what would it be? I went to the bathroom. When I came out he was standing right by the door. He grabbed me by the hair and assaulted my mouth with his tongue. He was a marvelous kisser. His tongue danced about mine in such a heady manner that I thought my knees were going to give out beneath me.

His bedroom wasn't far away. We fell onto his bed in a storm of kisses.

One third of participants in the Paris Report were submissive, one third were dominant, and one third switched back and forth between dominant and submissive roles.

—The Paris Report

Then, just as suddenly, he let me go, seeming to lose all interest in me. As he languorously went to pour himself another glass of wine, I stood up and tried to arrange my clothing and regain some sort of composure. I was slightly intoxicated, even without any wine, and quite bewildered. I drove home and collapsed into a deep sleep. It was the beginning of our tumultuous journey.

ILONA PARIS ON ACCEPTING YOUR KINK

People may be kinky in their twenties, when you are most experimental. You tend to put it aside when you marry, then, twenty years later, wind up on my couch in therapy because you can't stop thinking about it. But who ever said you can't enjoy your kink? Your mother? The church? The government? This is not about abuse—it's about having fun. Find your passion and free your spirit. Life is too hard not to enjoy yourself and the world you live in.

Shortly after that incident, Ivan sent me an e-mail with instructions for our next meeting.

Technically the focus here was called D/S—dominance and submission. I was to wear full makeup and a short black skirt with black pumps. I was to insert a pair of panties in my pussy prior to meeting him. I wasn't sure how to do this, so I practiced putting the panties up there beforehand. Of course, I was not to wear any panties on top of all this. When I arrived at his house, we went back to the deck. It was dusk, and he told me to lift my skirt and stand in front of him. He lived in a close-knit, family-oriented neighborhood. The houses were right on top of each other. You can imagine my shock at being displayed in public like this. I was disconcerted, and yet at the same time my cunt became wet and juicy. My nipples hardened through the tight little T-shirt I was wearing.

KINK AND THE LONG-TERM COUPLE

Kink can spice up a sagging relationship. Not only can it ignite nerve endings that you thought had maxed out years ago, it can also deepen a relationship and bring more trust and love between you. What goes on between the two of you, in an atmosphere of respect and mutual safety, can be playful, titillating, and inspiring. Doesn't this sound like something you want in your life? I know I do.

He made me sit opposite him and told me to spread my legs, exposing my pussy at all times. I was to be attentive to lighting his cigarette and placing the ashtray in front of him. This is the service aspect of D/S. Service could mean putting away the Dom's laundry, carrying the groceries, or wrapping meat for the freezer. For many submissives, this feels very fulfilling. Submission to another individual can actually bring about a deep peace, but for me it had the effect of fingernails on a chalkboard.

Still, Ivan was determined that I would be his submissive. He even collared me. Collaring is when someone puts a certain kind of necklace, or collar, around the submissive's neck, denoting

ADVANTAGES TO BEING SUBMISSIVE

- A release from the stresses of everyday life

- An adrenaline rush from totally letting go

- Freedom and empowerment

- A sense of redemption—you know how people in the Bible
  are always beating themselves to become cleansed of
  their sins?

- A sense of healing

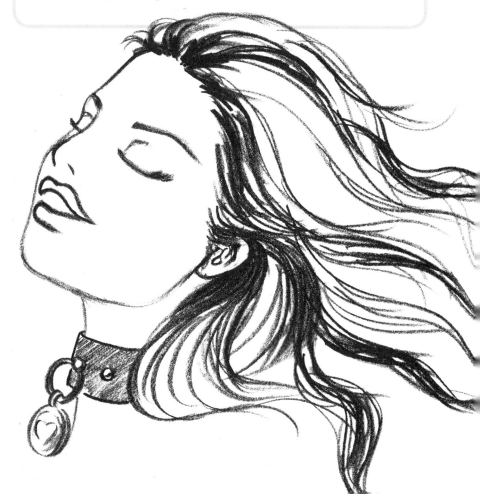

that he or she belongs to this person. The collar he gave me was a heavy metal ring held together by a metal lock. It looked like a piece of equipment from a construction site, but it obviously meant a great deal to him. He made me kneel at his feet with my head bowed as he placed it around my neck and locked it. It was uncomfortable and heavy. I didn't like it. I would have preferred a silver Tiffany necklace with a lock and key.

He sent me an e-mail listing the rules I was to live by. Whenever he asked me, "What is the bitch?" I was to respond by saying, "I am your shameless whore, Sir." He would then ask, "What kind of whore is the bitch?" I would respond by saying, "A cock-sucking, cunt-lapping, ass-fucked, come-drinking, piss-guzzling whore, Sir." I don't know about you, but so many compound words gave me a headache. At first blush, it seemed tawdry and off-putting. But then a funny thing happened. Because I wasn't used to it, being exposed to this vulgarity was kind of sexy. It was so different from anything I had encountered before that it put me in a different, more receptive place. I found it went straight to my cunt.

Surprisingly, I found Ivan to be an extremely giving person. A true Dom should be able to be a good mentor and to give in ways that are bursting with love, compassion, and understanding. Ivan could do this. He listened to my problems for hours and always tried to help me figure out a solution. We both had great senses of humor and enjoyed many sessions of gut-busting laughter. We adored snuggling together and I found great solace in having this huge man surround me with his arms and legs while I nestled in the warmth of that big chest. We did laundry, cooked, and went grocery shopping together. I was the focus of his world when we were together.

ILONA PARIS ON SUBMISSION

How do I become a sub(missive)?

First things first. You have to find out if you are submissive or not. In many cases you intuitively know: Like being gay or straight, it's something you feel in your gut. But like me, you may have to go through a trial period of trying things out, figuring out what you desire and need. Some people like to switch back and forth between dominant and submissive, but most people eventually become clear on which one they prefer. You may try being a sub and evolve into being dominant or vice versa. The most important thing is being true to yourself. Don't be afraid to give in to what feels right. You will feel more at peace with yourself and your life.

Will I have any say in what my dominant partner is doing?

Here's the surprising thing: the submissive is actually in control! It's the submissive who decides what can and can't be explored, sets the limits, and always retains the preemptive power to abort the session at any time by using a safe word. In that sense, the dominant is merely the facilitator, creating a situation wherein the submissive's fantasies can be explored. However, the dominant needs to have an intuition for when to push the envelope for the sub.

What if I just don't know which way to turn?

If you're hopelessly confused by all this, I have a one-word answer for you. "Surrender." The thing to keep in mind is that, like most of life, the choice of whether you turn out to be submissive or dominant is ultimately about intimacy and building relationships. You never know where you might meet someone or how it will evolve once you do. It can't be forced. You need to see what the universe provides you. You can optimize your chances by positioning yourself where like-minded people hang out, but you might find the relationship you need in your own living room over a glass of wine with someone. Relationships take work, compassion, and understanding—the same in this arena as in any other.

Ivan wanted me to write to him of my hungers. During the day at various intervals he wanted me to masturbate to near-orgasm for him. For me, this was extremely frustrating. Never deny me my orgasm! My personal credo is, the more orgasms the merrier. It gives the hair its shine, the step its bounce, the blood its song. I get squirmy just thinking about it.

Most people who visited the Fetish Flea Market reported earning a salary ranging from $55,000 to $100,000. —The Paris Report

But a lot of people love being sexually teased like this. In the D/S Scene, it shows a submissive's level of commitment and can be a powerful tool, creating great excitement and titillation. As I was to find out, it's fun to deny or delay another person's orgasm. Just don't delay or deny mine!

As you can probably guess, my soul began to rebel after a few months. I loved Ivan and wanted to work things out with him, but being a servant flew against my own empowerment as a woman. It made me extremely irritable, which led me to understand at last that I was not a submissive.

Ivan and I were together for a year. I became disenchanted. I started to see what was behind the curtain of the great Oz. He lived his life at the far end of the spectrum of alternative lifestyles—specifically the arena of polyamory, which is participation in multiple, simultaneous sexual relationships. He liked orgies, watching me with other men, and having me watch him with other women. I relished a good fuck as much as ever, but I experienced great jealousy in some of these situations. I found I didn't have the mental makeup to deal with polyamory. It pained me in a deep way that I didn't want to play around with.

VIOLENCE VS. ABUSE

Many people are under the false belief that sadomasochism is about violence and abuse. In her book, A Defense of Masochism, *Anita Phillips writes, "S&M practices are nothing like real violence. . . . In consensual sadomasochism the idea is to control pain for sexual purposes, [and] to stop when it goes beyond that limit. To equate the two is like comparing traffic noise to a sonata."*

We finally split. It took about eight months. I kept going back, and of course held on to the sex. He was a wonderful lover. He knew how to move that cock, which made it hard to give up. Also, if I broke up with Great White, would I be severing myself from the Scene? What would happen to me? Would I survive? Would I have any friends or connections to that world?

If only I knew then what a rich world of debauchery and exploration I was about to enter . . .

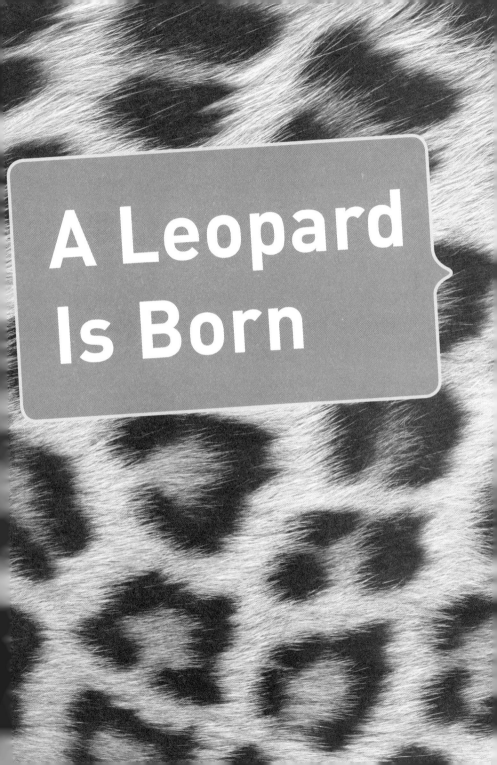

A Leopard
Is Born

Could I live this close to the
flame without getting singed?

The sight was as exquisite as a rare antique oil painting: a beautiful man standing in the middle of the room, totally naked. I stared transfixed at the rope, thick and white, wrapped around the man's helpless wrists. Beneath the black leather blindfold, his lips curled in an expression of pain mixed with pleasure as the Mistress, Lady Latex, added clothespin after clothespin to his cock and balls. Drops of sweat glistened on his skin under the pale light of a single golden candle. Quick: can you picture your partner in that position? Would you enjoy it?

This was my first exposure to what a Mistress actually did. I knew for sure I wasn't a sub. But did I have it in me to become a professional dominatrix, trained by a honey-maned blonde named Lady Latex?

It sounded good on paper: The money was decent and the hours were even better, allowing me time to continue my practice as a sexual therapist. But what appealed to me most was that it fleshed out, as it were, the academic textbooks I'd been studying all these years. Here was my chance to put all those dry case studies of sexual deviancy to the test, to see it up close and personal, in all its glorious 3D. I felt that the clinical world misinterpreted this lifestyle. What clinician actually went into the dungeon to become that which she studied? How could it not help me be a more understanding clinician?

And yes, I have to admit: the perversity of it appealed to me, too. I liked the idea of working a vanilla job by day and a whacked-out job by night. It was wild, it was crazy, and it put me close to the flame, where I had always lived in some way or another. But could I do it this time without being singed?

HOW TO BE SEXUALLY MISCHIEVOUS

1. Read this book.

2. Be open and creative.

3. Go with what intrigues you and catches your attention.

4. If you find yourself thinking or fantasizing about it, try it.

5. Anything goes, but remember: Always be safe, sane, and consensual.

I'd known about sadomasochism for years, of course. I'd studied the classic theorems of Emil Durkheim and read the new theories by Charles Moser and leather writings by Pat Califa. I knew by heart the quotation from Lynn Cowan: "the masochist . . . comes to terms with the greatest opposites of our existence." All this and more I knew in my head: that some people prefer to be submissive or dominant all the time, while others like to switch back and forth, playing a submissive role one day and a dominant one the next. That sadomasochism doesn't always involve whips and chains; it can be remarkably sensual and soft, involving little more than blindfolding your partner and running rabbit fur over his body. That not everyone is interested in pain (inflicting or receiving); some just want to be tied up and tickled, or be tortured with ice cubes, or enjoy the high they get from ordering their partners around. That like any specialty, it's as varied as the people who practice it.

But it was one thing to know this stuff intellectually, and entirely another to witness it for myself. And in such a setting! It gave me a chuckle to think that such an exotic, feared, and misunderstood practice as S&M was being practiced not in a rococo

"Perfection for a naked pleasure slave must be yielding to the most extreme punishments. The slave spiritualizes these ordeals, no matter how crude and painful. And all the torments of the village, even more than the more decorous humiliations of the castle, tumble fast one upon the other in an endless current of excitement. . . . And who understands power, worships it, more than those who have had it?"
— *A. N. Roquelaure*, Beauty's Punishment

castle garret somewhere in southern France but in the basement of a nondescript Rhode Island ranch house with a white picket fence and avocado-green appliances, converted into a modern-day S&M dungeon.

WHAT'S YOUR FANTASY?

Are you a severe schoolmarm, a latex or leather diva, a sexy nurse? Do you want your look to be severe, sexy, commanding, buxom, ice queen? Ask your partner what turns him or her on and enjoy yourself.

My initiation into dominatrix life had actually begun two weeks earlier at Kinky Folks, a Rhode Island club for people with unusual sexual proclivities. I was invited to the cigarette smoke–filled hall of a VFW post after hours to give a guest lecture, and had been mesmerized by the sight of male and female flesh gleaming under a spotlight. Could I really enter into this electrifying Scene—and make good money to boot? Weighing the risk to my therapeutic career and mental sanity, I felt that I could keep both in balance for a period of time. I had made the acquaintance of Lady Latex, and one thing led to another. She had agreed to take me under her wing to become a full-fledged dominatrix with my own clientele.

I had a lot to learn.

Lady Latex set me straight about some of the basics from the get-go. There was a world of difference between a Domme and a prostitute, she stressed. All those "jobs"—blow jobs, hand jobs, and the like—were out of the question. So was most every other kind of sexual contact, in the ordinary sense of the phrase, between the Domme and her client. In fact, the only part of Lady Latex's body he or she could touch, and only with permission, were her feet—which became highly sexualized as a result. (This can differ from Mistress to Mistress, but it was the rule I preferred.) But she warned me never to forget that male clients tended to be intrinsically stronger than female Dommes, and that I had always to remain firmly in control, lest the client turn on me. That's where

THE APPEARANCE FACTOR

One thing I didn't have to learn was how to look.

It was apparent to me from the outset that, if clients were prepared to pay a great deal of money in exchange for our specialized services, we had to be prepared to play our part with all the flair at our disposal. The fantasy they were buying was as important as the activity itself. Dramatic makeup and a natural sense of grace provided a good amount of the smoke and mirrors, while education and training provided the craftsmanship.

But it's the wardrobe that separates the women from the girls. Fetish clothes create the illusion of power, strength, and sublime beauty. Don't scrimp in this department, because people in the Scene judge you by the type and quality of the clothes you wear. I mean, for God's sake, cut out the tags in your thongs, ladies.

One outfit I like is a pair of black patent-leather hot pants with a matching buckled vest. I wear a black garter belt, black stockings, and a pair of black leather platform boots that lace all the way up the front.

Another elegant piece I love is a Catherine Coatney item

the infamous orgasmic "release" came in—as much self-protection as anything else.

I had to be a little like a lion tamer, she said—I could put my head in the beast's mouth, but only if I was sure it wasn't going to bite.

Continuing her crash course into the kind of real-life reality I couldn't get from classrooms, Lady Latex tried to allay my fears about this unknown world. She was a remarkably intuitive person,

that is simply delicious. Coatney is a famous California-based designer of fetishwear whose designs I find to be unfailingly stylish and sophisticated. The outfit is similar to a full-length girdle top, or maybe a girdlette, with patent leather down the front and garters at the bottom. The back is a sheer black girdle-like material that just covers my rump. I wear it with a little patent-leather thong underneath and let my cheeks peek out. I'm so partial to this item, in fact, that it was the one I chose to wear for my first photo shoot, which was featured in Domination Directory International *magazine (DDI).*

When I'm in a festive mood, I slip into a full-length black latex gown complete with thin gold straps with buckles that come to a V in the front of the bodice. It has a slit that comes all the way up to my thigh. I wear it with black fishnets and six-inch fetish shoes in black patent leather with straps down the sides. A pair of full-length black latex gloves complete the effect I want, which is that of a supreme goddess.

Oh, and please make sure your latex is fully shined to a high gloss. On your knees, slave!

ILONA PARIS ON DOMINANCE

How do I know if I'm dominant?

Dominance is a pretty fancy word for a pretty basic condition. It is something that already exists deep inside you; something you were born with that you have the ability to tap under the right circumstances. It's nothing, in other words, that you need to dream up or put on. It's something you have to reach down and locate within yourself. If it doesn't feel right, maybe it's not you. But if the following sounds familiar, my friend, well . . .

At eight years old, you tie your pesky little neighbor to a tree and throw skunk cabbage at him while calling him names (I actually did this). At twelve, you belt your best friend because she talked behind your back at lunch. And feel pretty good about it afterwards. And there's you at fifteen, babysitting for the brat next door and ordering him to stand still and not move a muscle.

What if my partner doesn't want to be dominated?

I see this all the time in therapy. I encourage couples to go slow, to try something very gentle to begin with. Maybe it's as vanilla as a sexy backrub—one during which your lover is not allowed to move or make noise or you will stop. The next week have him or her flip over for a "front rub," with the same rules, plus a side of light bondage. Maybe his or her hands are tied to the headboard. Or try to find a scene in which he or she would like to be a submissive. If it's really not working, try trading places on different nights.

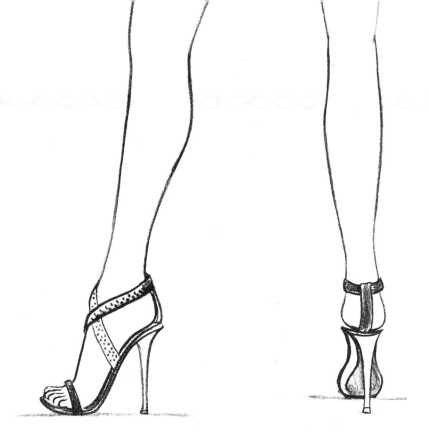

What if I'm not sure?

Most likely you know, but you may have to dig down and allow your true sexual self out of the box that is "normal" society. Dominance is an attitude. A mind-set. An outlook. One that has perhaps served you well in life, maybe without your even knowing it. That has gotten you, in fact, where you are today. It's a certain tone of voice, an expression you wear, the posture you hold.

Polite but firm. Commanding but humane. In control. And in the company of another consenting adult, Instantly Sexy. Eternally Erotic. Just thinking about the word makes me wet. Take control—at least once—and see if you don't feel the same way.

and correctly sensed that as a human being I had my fears as much as anyone else. And boy, did I. Would this open up a can of worms in my own makeup? I had a lot of trust issues and didn't like the idea of giving someone else control over me. If I allowed myself to explore this part of my personality, would people make fun of me? Would they think I was a terrible person? Would they take advantage of me somehow—financially or personally? The world could be a hard place, I knew. I didn't want to revisit the place where I sometimes felt like a vulnerable little girl under attack. But then, we were talking about my taking control. And wouldn't this escapade be more fun than almost anything I'd ever done?

SELF-DISCOVERY AND S&M

When I was initially attracted to S&M, it was my kink gene ringing loud and clear. It has led me like a magnet on a path of self-discovery the likes of which I never would have imagined. From the beginning, I didn't want S&M just to provoke my nerve endings. I wanted to use S&M to deepen my humanity and maybe even enliven my spirituality, if that were possible. The truth is, I just had no idea what unbelievable doors it would open.

A top-notch dominatrix, I learned, is an artisan. There is a deep beauty to her practice. She appreciates the aesthetic of a well-executed "tortoiseshell body harness," such as the one introduced by the Japanese fetish diva Midori, and understands how a client might spend an hour in abject devotion to a woman's well-turned ankle (I have a beautiful tattoo on mine—a bird of paradise in purple, orange, and green). But mostly I had to learn the etiquette. It is of paramount importance, for instance, that a dominatrix maintain respect for her client, even as she is "abusing" him or her. I had to be exquisitely attuned to his needs, with empathy and the ability to read and judge my submissive's reactions and take him to

the place he wanted to go. A person who chooses to be a dominant must possess the ability to exhibit great compassion and cruelty at the same time. A great Mistress or Master will instill a sense of mentorship and help the person to grow.

So I was more than ready to begin my first session as a dominatrix-in-training. I had

> A predilection for S&M does seem to exist and appears in childhood. Fifty percent of people in the study had their first kinky thoughts between the ages of five and twelve.
> —*The Paris Report*

driven down to this residential neighborhood in my Beetle named Shirley, and had parked in Lady Latex's driveway. I was dressed carefully in a very tight pair of black Levi's and a slinky black button-down shirt. My fire-engine red toenails poked out from my gold metallic high-heeled sandals. After a few preliminaries (touching up our makeup in her pink bathroom and reviewing protocol), Lady Latex and I descended a set of shaky wooden stairs to the basement dungeon.

Outside the dungeon door was a heart-shaped wooden box into which the client had placed his "tribute"—$250 in nice, clean bills. Well, that worked for me. Next to the box Lady Latex had set out her business cards, elegant little affairs that simply stated, "Lady Latex," with a phone number underneath. She carried a plastic cup of water with a straw. This, she indicated, was for the slave in case he became dehydrated. Heaven forbid he dry up on us while we tortured him. Oh yeah, this was gonna be the real deal. The little bit of intimidation I was feeling was more than offset by the fascination I felt in the face of the growing mystery.

Inside, the air was heavy. Everything was black: the walls, the ceiling, the rubber tiles on the floor. Under the light of one flickering candle, there were hoods made of leather, metal, rubber, and more black leather. A row of paddles hung across one of the walls, and an assortment of floggers—featuring soft, flat strands of leather—were hanging by chains from the ceiling. An umbrella stand was filled with canes and riding crops. Lengths of rope hung from hooks, all soft and pliable from the washer/dryer treatment Lady Latex gave them (which also helped keep everything sterilized—a big difference between the pros and the beginners). Inside a dramatic black lacquer cabinet I spied alcohol, needles, Wartenberg wheels, and dildos of every shape and size—and I do mean *every*: purple popsicles, dancing dolphins, and giant creamsicles that vibrated. It was a candy store for the perverted.

The slave himself had been transformed from a rather normal-looking thirty-eight-year-old computer geek in gold-rimmed glasses, jeans, and a white polo shirt, into a naked slave making an offering of his quivering flesh. He had stashed his clothes in a closet and submitted to being tied. Lady Latex was clear that you should always tie down a new client until you know for sure he isn't dangerous. With his hands bound behind his back, he was on his knees in front of a throne that instilled a chilling mix of fear and awe—a purple velvet structure with heavy walnut wood and black leather arm pads. In the candlelight, his skin was smooth, and his

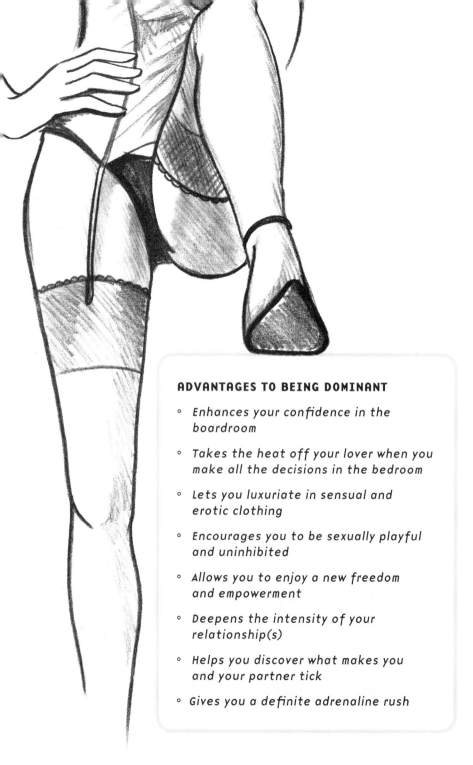

ADVANTAGES TO BEING DOMINANT

- *Enhances your confidence in the boardroom*

- *Takes the heat off your lover when you make all the decisions in the bedroom*

- *Lets you luxuriate in sensual and erotic clothing*

- *Encourages you to be sexually playful and uninhibited*

- *Allows you to enjoy a new freedom and empowerment*

- *Deepens the intensity of your relationship(s)*

- *Helps you discover what makes you and your partner tick*

- *Gives you a definite adrenaline rush*

muscles subtly rippled beneath its surface. His buttocks were just waiting to be kneaded. I felt a smile beginning.

So when Lady Latex asked if I was ready to play, I narrowed my eyes and surveyed my prey. "Mmm, let me see if I can raise his temperature a bit."

Ever so gently, Lady Latex tipped a candle so a sizzling trail of wax dribbled down the slave's backside. As he bit his lip and whimpered, Lady Latex put the candle down and slid his blindfold on. She grabbed him by the hair and yanked him to his feet, ordering him to spread his legs wide, wider, *wider!* Then she handed me a flogger with a silver filigree handle and three feet of silky blond horsehair.

How can I convey what it felt like to hear the words: "He's all yours"?

THE ART OF PREPARATION

Getting ready for a date with your lover can be its own form of foreplay. Enjoy the sensation of pulling on a pair of stockings and clasping them to a garter. Linger in the door of your closet, imagining which outfit would turn him on most. Does he like vintage hose? Slutty heels and thigh-highs? Or what about a spectacular lingerie outfit? I once knew a man who swooned at the sight of a French twist, glasses, and a black suit with matching stilettos. Choose your weapons, girls, and go for it!

I sauntered over like a runway model and took up position in front of the slave, who hung his head in quaking anticipation of what was to come. His cock, decorated with clothespins, was so hard it must have been difficult for him to breathe. I started slowly, getting him used to me, as if I were training a horse. I began flogging him almost lovingly between his legs, watching the horsehair slide between the crack of his ass and over his balls. I loved the way the muscles in his buttocks and back twitched each time I did it.

After a minute of this warm-up, I untied his wrists and gave him permission to kiss my feet. I stood with my hands on my hips, pointed my toes and looked down my nose at him. His rock-solid cock bounced up and down with excitement, pulsing with his heartbeat as he craned to do my bidding. I felt his warm breath on my toes, then his lips brushed lightly over them, soft and sweet. "Hmm," I thought, "I could get used to this."

I was amazed at how right it felt, deep down within my bones, as though I'd been searching for this all my life.

One hour later, Lady Latex handed me a wad of cash. Not bad for an hour's work. I gave Lady Latex a peck on the cheek and hopped into Shirley. I had agreed to meet my best friend, a big queen named Teddy, at the Jackie Kennedy exhibit being held in the Kennedy Library in Dorchester, featuring all her stunning out-fits designed by Oleg Cassini. I could hardly wait. I loved the idea of beating a naked man one minute and ogling Jackie O.'s threads the next. I had packed a ham and cheese sandwich for the ride and nibbled on it while I pondered what I should use for a name. How about Lady Leopard? Not only did I have a thing for leopard skin, I also believed a leopard possessed qualities of agility, strength, and feline beauty, as well as the ability to attack and kill with incredible speed. Yes, this would be my name: Lady Leopard. As I zoomed along the highway, nibbling my sandwich, I knew I was in for one hell of a ride.

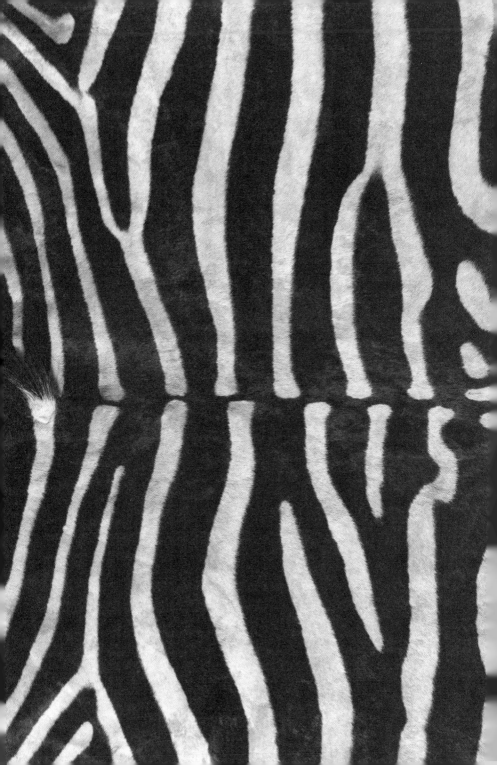

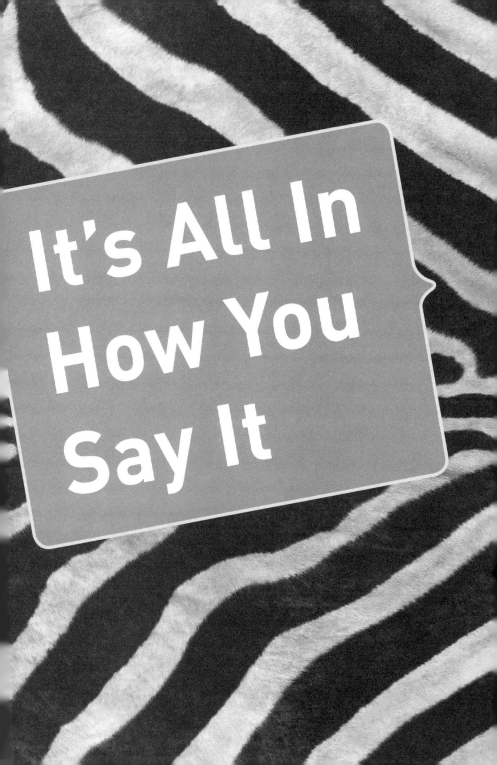

It's All In How You Say It

Are they dirty words – or passwords to a hotter sex life?

Words! When they're the right ones, they can set the libido ablaze. I found that out when I got involved with a smooth-talking radio host whose business was words, words, words.

Radio Man was alluring due to his star power, and also because he was married. Doing it on the sly with him made it extra exciting, like we had to sneak around and whisper all the time. But the things we whispered about! We used dirtier words than I had ever used in my life. We threw all self-consciousness to the wind and said every nasty thing we could think of. I loved what he said and how he said it. His voice was rich and smooth as heavy cream. I liked to bathe in the sound of it while he held me in his arms, feeling the vibrations through my skin.

Radio Man's words transfixed me in every medium, whether it was via e-mail, instant message, or text message. Sometimes I would turn on his station as I got into my car in the morning just to start my day with him. The smooth timbre of his vocal tool took me over the edge.

Instead of getting bored with each other, which is always the potential downside of any relationship, our lovemaking became more open and creative over time because of the trust between us. It became my goal to excite this man out of his mind. His radio station was only fifteen minutes from my apartment. I had transformed my apartment into a dungeon complete with wardrobe, bondage bed, floor-to-ceiling mirror, tool box, and so on (see "The Nitty Gritty" for the Full Monty). I liked to be ready for him when he came off the air. I created outrageous theme outfits for his arrival. One day I wore an Oriental red satin corset, which he had bought me, with a matching G-string and vintage stockings.

Make your voice sultry and elegant.
Nothing is better than dishing out the dirt
with a graceful mouth.

Another day I wore nothing but a gold chain around my waist and a pair of clear Lucite heels. I put my hands on either side of the doorway, with my legs seductively crossed, and stood at the end of the hallway waiting for him to walk in the door. He'd been emceeing that day for a big golf tournament, and walked in reeking of cigars. He wanted to take a shower. This nude goddess is standing there, and he wants to take a shower? Then he decided to shave, not once but twice. Then he brushed his teeth and gargled. Then he blow-dried his hair. At that point I was lying on the couch reading my third Victoria's Secret catalog. We both cracked up.

Usually, though, we started in with the dirty talk the second he walked through the door. "Fuck me. I need you to fuck me . . . "

Sometimes we would make it to the bedroom, but usually we couldn't get past the living room. That's how dazzling it was between us.

WORDS FROM THE MASTER:
"Th'art good cunt, though, are'nt ter?
Best bit o' cunt left on earth . . ."
"What is cunt?" she said.
"An' doesn't ter know? Cunt! It's thee
down theer; an' what I get when I'm
i'side thee, and what tha gets when
I'm i' side thee . . . "
"Cunt! It's like fuck then."
"Nay nay! Fuck's only what you do.
Animals fuck. But cunt's a lot more
than that. It's thee, dost see: an'
tha'rt a lot besides an animal, are
n't ter?—even ter fuck! Cunt! Eh,
that's the beauty o' thee, lass!"
—*D.H. Lawrence*, Lady Chatterley's Lover

Then one glorious day he decided to amp it up a notch. He put me on the radio with him for a live interview. I had done several radio interviews before in my capacity as a "sexpert who specializes in alternative erotic lifestyles"—and I'd been told I gave good radio.

Our conversation follows:

Radio Man: *Ms. Paris, I'm wondering right off the top—with the experience you've garnered in your practice, why do you think it is that men are so attracted to phone sex? Are the reasons varied as to why men do this?*

Ms. Paris: *We have five senses, and hearing is one of them. Erotically, we all love to satisfy our senses where we are excited to a point of release. Talking sexy on the phone, or elsewhere for that matter, can stimulate that large organ known as the brain.*

Radio Man: *So it's sort of like providing gas for your car?*

Ms. Paris: *That's one aspect of it. Sure.*

Radio Man: *Ms. Paris, do you think a man is perverted because he likes to have phone sex?*

Ms. Paris: *Randomly calling people with dirty phone calls is not healthy. But when two people voluntarily decide to excite each other using their ears and voices, now there you have something very hot. That is definitely healthy and can be very creative.*

Radio Man: *Do you think it's normal?*

Ms. Paris: *Well, what one person thinks is normal, another does not. People have been using sexy talk as part of their erotic lives since the beginning of time. In fact, it is rumored that Adam and Eve started it.*

Radio Man: *Ms. Paris, is it the thrill? Is it not being seen that makes it so arousing? So the imagination is free to wander as much as it wants?*

Ms. Paris: *All of the above. Every one of those details can be extremely suggestive to the couple engaging in phone sex, especially if both of them are verbally dexterous. Aural sex can be the best thing in the world . . .*

Radio Man: *Oral sex? Well, sure, if you want to talk about oral sex, who doesn't like that?*

Ms. Paris: *I believe you misheard me. I said aural, not oral. Aural, as in hearing. Using the right words in the right way. People need to learn the words that turn each other on, and to use their voices to say those words in the best way.*

Radio Man: *You mean how you regulate your voice could turn someone on?*

Ms. Paris: *Absolutely. It's all in what you say and how you say it . . .*

Radio Man: *Well, we are out of time, but we certainly must have you back.*

Words are only half of the aural appeal.
The other half is breathing. Try breathing softly and
watch what effect this has on your honey.
Try breathing fast. Try catching your breath, then
letting it out in a stuttering fashion.
Hold your breath, and then expel it hard.
So many people are afraid to make noise. Let it rip.

Cut to fifteen minutes later. My legs were tense with anticipation. I felt that stirring inside where I just wanted to be filled by him. Our own aural factor had worked once again between the two of us, this time on the radio in front of thousands of people. Aural stimulation combined with exhibitionism is a tantalizing cocktail. It was like we'd been flirting even while being so careful not to. We'd gone public but stayed private at the same time, flaunting our sex life before the world even while we weren't breathing a word. Truly a game of on-air tightrope. I was ready to come like a fucking fire engine. My bells were ringing loud and clear.

TRY THIS

- *When you are at a dinner party, walk up to your lover and simply state, "I want to fuck you." Then walk away.*

- *Call your loved one during the day while he or she is at work. Tell him or her what you would like to do to his cock or her pussy and then hang up.*

- *Stressed while on a business trip? Pick up the phone and tell your lover exactly what you would like to do him. Masturbate with each other. Uh huh.*

- *Try talking into your partner's underwear and watch the cock factor come alive!*

- *Kick up the heat while doing the evening dishes. Sneak up behind your partner, slowly cover his eyes, and talk into his ear about how much you want to fuck him up the ass. Your dishes will be nice and clean.*

- *Hide scarves under the bed. When your lover least expects it, tie him or her to the bedposts and use a blindfold as well. Whisper that a stranger is coming through the door to fuck one of you. Can you take it from there?*

I reached into my workman's tool chest filled with erotic wear and pulled out a pair of vintage thigh-highs and nothing else. I put on five-inch black stilettos courtesy of Ivan. I looked in the floor-length mirrors and felt this would do. There is nothing like lascivious simplicity. In no time, I could see Radio Man through the window, striding from his gold SUV across the street to my

ILONA PARIS ON THE ALLURE OF AURAL SEX

As I said, aural sex has doubtless been around since Adam and Eve. In fact, I believe that Eve got so excited one day she just had to pick up that apple and bite into something so she didn't hurt Adam.

And it's been riveting people ever since.

Face it: there is something extremely stimulating about fantasizing with the visual while listening to the audio. Look at all the phone ads in the backs of newspapers. It's no coincidence that this is such a big industry in America. Given how big it is, and what an important role it plays in everyone's libido, don't you think it behooves us to learn to train our voices for utmost sexual effect?

It's helpful for everyone—not just people with sex on the brain, like you and me, but everyone—to think of his or her voice as a musical instrument. Instead of squawking out a command, learn to make it sultry. Instead of shouting, think about how much power there is in whispering. Lowering your voice can convey extraordinary authority. Learn to listen to your voice and regulate it, learn how to control it just as if you were using a stick shift in a car. You want to steer your voice so you can go fast on a highway, go slow in an alleyway, and sometimes cut loose in an abandoned parking lot. You want to be able to learn how to shift your vocal faculties so that you are free to experience your erotica with both control and abandon. Now doesn't that sound like fun?

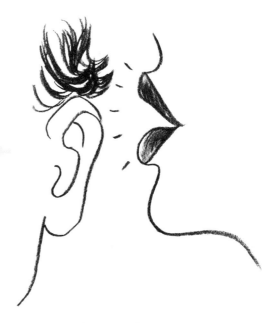

How to Start

It's essential that you hear how your voice sounds to others. Listen to it on a tape recorder or on a message you've left on your phone. Practice reading something sexy when you are home alone, or maybe have your honey nearby and gauge how all this reading is affecting him. Hard or soft? Alluring or off-putting? Figure it out, darlings.

Imitate speakers or singers you admire. I don't mean go to the shower and belt out the Top 40. I mean notice women who seem to be in control of their voices. Think Lauren Bacall. Think Sharon Stone or Susan Sarandon. Think Nora Jones. Slow down. Enunciate your words. Play with the volume control of your voice. It's not an on/off switch, loud or quiet; it's a dial that you can tune up or tune down, a continuum. Play with all the varying levels of volume in between loud and quiet, between vibrating and breathless. Understand the command you can have if you learn to modulate that wonderful instrument in your throat.

And always: Watch the effect it has on people. Experiment.

door. As soon as the doorbell rang, I threw my arms around my big famous radio interviewer. I curled a leg around his knees. Our tongues met and I went to a place that was so comfortable and delirious for me. All the pent-up desire that had been building on air was finally going to be released, and I could feel his cock immediately spring to attention. I slid my hand inside his trousers, grabbed all eight inches, and slipped to my knees. "Cock," I said in my sultriest voice. "I want your cock," and looked directly into his eyes.

"I like what you say and how you say it," Radio Man said.

"Cock," I said again, reaching out and placing it in my mouth. "Cock, cock, cock, cock . . ."

Don't think of them as dirty words.
Think of them as passwords. Passwords to a harder
cock and a moister cunt.

His baby blues were hypnotized as he watched my mouth saying the words while I licked my private lollipop. "Cock, you cock you, you big cock . . ."

"Mouth," he groaned. "Your mouth on my dick, your lips on my dick . . ."

I could feel my juices rejoicing as I heard him describe what my mouth was doing to him. He was verbally dexterous, and other kinds of dexterous, too.

"I'm your big boy."

I inhaled the scent of baby powder. Jesus, I loved that cock!

"Put it in me now."

His balls were ample in size, and I lightly scratched my nails behind them. "I want to hear my balls slapping up against your ass," he said.

"That can be arranged, but lick me first," I breathed. "Lick me, lick me, lick me, lick me . . ."

He immediately got down on his knees and used that magnificent tongue to lick my pussy. Once again, I was surprised at how warm and smooth it felt on my clit. It was perfect. I sighed outwardly and my head naturally fell back. Within a second I knew I needed him inside of me.

REMEMBER THIS!

Don't feel guilty or prudish if trash talkin' doesn't do it for you. Some people find it a turn-on and some people don't. Some people like it as a steady diet, some like it during foreplay only, and some don't like it anytime. There's nothing wrong with not enjoying any particular aspect of sexual mischief. I myself found that certain topics were a turn-off to me. Instead of getting down on yourself for not liking something, find something that hits your hot spot. God knows, there's enough to go around!

The floor-to-ceiling mirror was made for this kind of fucking. I loved looking at the intensity of his face as he slid his shaft inside me. Most of the time he was busy watching himself in the act, a typical man: he loved the visual. But the aural pleasure was there, too, now mostly in the form of his growling. And me growling back. As we went wild—fucking every which way, in and out, up and down—we growled like a couple of bears in the woods.

Radio Man could never take much of this before he would jump back in between my legs and give me the best tongue job a woman has ever had. He was a force of nature when it came to eating pussy! I loved looking at the top of his head and those ocean-blue eyes that glittered with concentration. He had this way of twirling his tongue around my pearl with just the right pressure. Men have a habit of using too much pressure. You need to be soft and warm, and swirl, boys, swirl!

Ahhh, this felt so good. All the passions we'd been forced to stifle came roiling out like thunder from on high. He knew exactly what to do with my clitoris, and sucked it with just the right pressure to make me have my first orgasm. Talk about dirty talk! I was shouting out a blue streak of obscenities as electric rods of energy shot through my body, making me scream and growl all at the same time.

And then the *coup de grace*: he started speaking right into my pussy lips. He kept his lips just perfectly over the area, warm and vibrating. "Pussy," he was saying, over and over. I focused and started to feel the warm vibrations emanating through my lips and then my loins. He had pulsed enough and the tsunami of orgasm was reaching the shore. Oh, fuck! He knew his cue and plunged deeply inside of me. He almost scared me—he was so big and came at me with such a ferocity I thought I would split in half. As far as I'm concerned, that's all a woman wants: a warm, silky tongue and then a nice, plunging fat cock. And all the time he kept talking with that filthy mouth of his. "Whose cock is this?" he asked. "Mine, it belongs to me," I answered. "Fuck me, give me that cock. My cock."

Saying this always brought him close to the edge. He flipped me over on top of him.

An advanced sexual vocabulary is a true asset,
but what's even better is the ability to be explicit.
The more explicit the better. Don't be shy:
nothing turns a man on more than a sweet little
mouth saying words that are absolutely filthy.

"Take this, you fucker," I growled. "You fat cock, you."

I grabbed his hands as he slowly and gloriously filled me to the top. I closed my eyes as he took his thumb and rubbed my slippery clit to the point where I was ready to explode. I sat all the way down and rubbed my pubic bone against him. I felt the heat rising and then gave way to a glorious eruption. Another deep growl rose from my throat as I fell over and bit his ear. He started screaming as he was coming. I kept growling, "Fuck me, give me your come, fuck me, give me your come." This drove the man into such a frenzy I thought he was going to rip my pussy apart before he came inside me for a long, long, long, long time.

"There it is, your come."

Silence. Silence at last. The words seemed to hang in the air as the bright sunlight streamed in on us from the bay windows. We looked down our bodies at all the carnage. We just giggled at the sight. We did what we always did after having sex: rolled over in a spoon position and just enjoyed the feel of each other quietly.

At last he murmured in my ear, "You're right, Ms. Paris."

"About what, sir?"

A beat.

"Aural sex can be the best thing in the world."

EXTRA! EXTRA! PHONE SEX!

As a dominatrix of many dimensions, it was not uncommon for me to conduct phone sessions. People sent me $100 in advance, and we set up a time for a half-hour session on the phone. This worked out well, because I could sit in my leopard-skin thermal pajamas and not have to spend time applying makeup or squirming into latex. I could sit back like I was the Queen of Sheba and drive some submissive man into a tizzy.

Corey, a high-powered stockbroker for Paine Webber, was a favorite phone sub of mine who adored female supremacy. Every month he sent me his tribute, and we set up a time for his session. For twenty-four hours prior to his session, he would have to keep a red ribbon tied tightly in a bow around his cock. "You are not to touch yourself," I told him in a firm, strict voice.

"Yes, Mistress," he replied.

The moment came for him to call me. "Hello, slut," I said. "Did you touch yourself?"

"No, Mistress."

"Good boy. Are you in your office on your knees?"

"Yes, Mistress."

"At Paine Webber? Hah!"

"Yes, Mistress."

"Would you like a little Paine to make up for all the people you bilked out of their life savings today?" (I had no idea whether he bilked anyone or not, but I so enjoyed tormenting the poor man.)

"Please, Mistress."

I then took him through a little scene in which I greeted him at the door. I described the latex outfit that I might be wearing. I told him I would have him strip naked in front of me because he was nothing but a little worm worthy only of sniveling around in the dirt. I told him how I would make him crawl before a group of women. Each one would make him suck her toes and then spank him. Then I would fuck him with a dildo.

"And you will thank me, worm!" I screamed.

"Yes, Mistress. May I have another, Mistress?" he whispered into the phone.

I could tell this guy was in a state.

"Would you like to come, you sniveling piece of scum?" I hollered.

I could hear him wanking his weenie. He was doing it real fast.

"Come for me," I ordered.

And come he did.

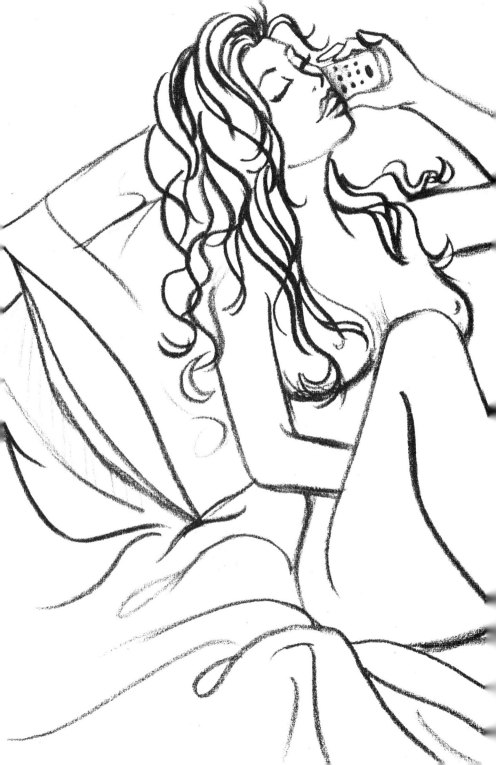

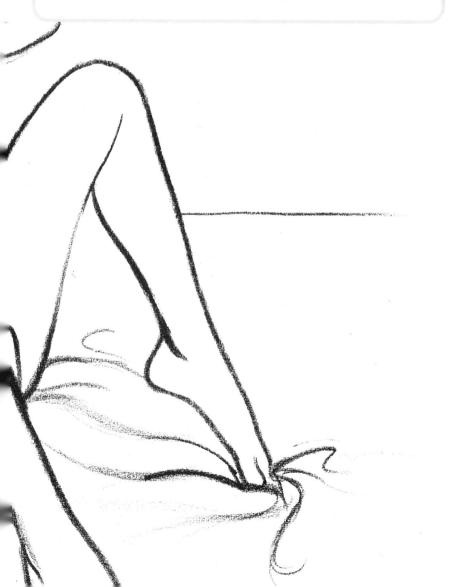

TIPS FOR BETTER PHONE SEX

The most important factor in devising your plan of approach when having phone sex is to know beforehand what your partner's hot button is. Does he go crazy at the thought of your getting it on with another woman or man, right in front of him? Figure that out and you're golden.

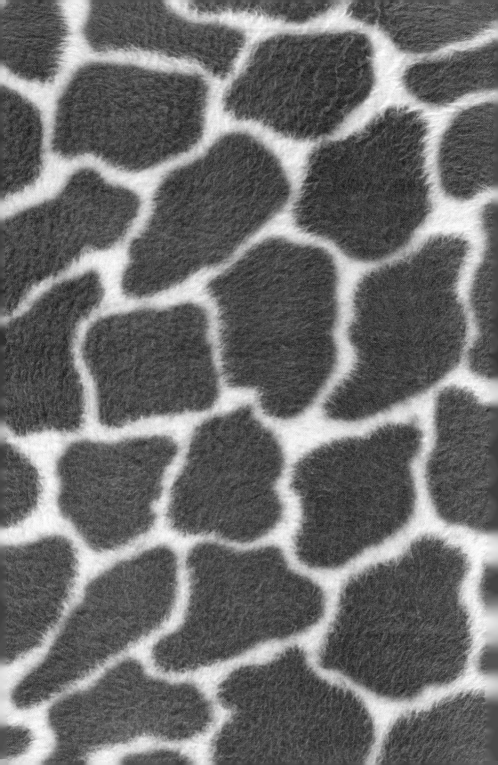

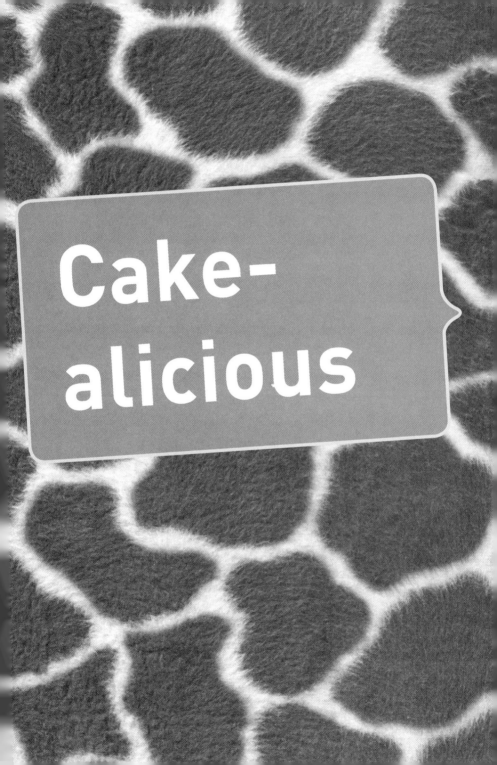

Cake-alicious

A kitchen quickie.

This'll just take a minute . . .

It is, after all, about a quickie.

You probably don't think of cake and sexual mischief in the same breath, but I have to get this off my chest. Quite literally.

I had always wanted to have a lover who could somehow combine my passion for food with passion for sex, and I found one in Radio Man. Radio Man fancied himself a connoisseur in the kitchen as much as the bedroom, and was into both interests as much as I was. He even understood my ultimate food fantasy, which I shared with him one day at a restaurant: that I would love to sit on a cake. Radio Man almost choked on his French fry. Raising his hand he had croaked, "Sign me up." I could always count on my partner in crime.

I thought he'd forgotten about it, though, until my birthday. I had gone out to dinner with friends and gotten home about midnight. No sooner had I waltzed in my door, when the phone rang. "May I come by?" I was never one to turn down that voice, oozing with sex.

Five minutes later the doorbell rang. There was Radio Man, with a large white box from Daniel's Bakery tied up in a string. "Remember when you mentioned sitting on a cake?" he asked with a wink.

I gasped. Was my secret wish about to come true? With a wicked little smile I pulled the string. There in front of me was the most luscious white iced cake in the world, a confectionery delight with succulent red strawberries encircling its top, waiting to be devoured. Radio Man grabbed one strawberry and popped it in my mouth. I squealed in delight.

There is nothing as delicious as jumping into the reality of one's fantasy. This was it. We carried the cake into the kitchen, where we placed my pink yoga mat on the floor. I placed the box of cake on top of the mat and opened the white cardboard flaps so the sides were splayed wide and flat. I turned around and prepared for my historic descent, slowly lowering my derriere onto the creamy whipped confection.

"Yow!" I screamed, rising at once. It was a chilly evening and the cake had been outside too long. However, I collected myself for another attempt. Nothing was going to stop me now.

Imagine being totally nude and sitting back into a luscious cake with the whipped cream slithering up between your thighs and pussy, then squishing your derriere so that you become one with the cake. The effect would be similar to a little piglet rolling around in mud with supreme happiness. The sensation of such a delightful concoction oozing in and out of me was almost other-worldly. The cold creaminess of my culinary pillow reached out and grabbed my clit, making it shudder. I threw my head back and laughed in delight. This was just too marvelously decadent.

EVERYDAY IS SOMEBODY'S BIRTHDAY

Why wait till your own birthday? Any day you and your honey choose, go out and bring home a slice of cake to celebrate. Make sure it's one with lots and lots of frosting. When you get home, lie in a prone position on the bed and order your lover to squish the cake into your pussy. He then must eat, lick, slurp, nibble, and otherwise ingest the cake right out of your privates. Wasn't this what Marie Antoinette really meant when she said, "Let them eat cake"?

I lay back and spread my thighs open. Radio Man quickly assumed his position on his knees between my legs. He smushed his face into my pussy and came up covered in whipped cream. I reached down and grabbed his head, bringing it to my mouth, and kissed him as deeply as was humanly possible. Nothing is better than letting go fully. It is so freeing and so wonderfully enveloping. I had become one with the whipped cream and strawberries. My taste buds and pussy were now singing the same song of sweet ecstasy. I had flown to another planet and was flying with Radio Man in our own private orbit.

I licked his face until I was satisfied that he was properly cleaned up. Then he dove in again to start licking my clit with its whipped-cream topping. It must have tasted similar to a clit short-cake—all berries and cream. He swirled his wonderful tongue around with a creamy flourish. I grabbed a handful of cake and smeared it all over Radio Man's great big chest, then over mine. I rubbed my breasts against his pecs and they slid together like velvet balloons. He stood above me with his rock-solid cock, which had never looked tastier. God, I loved that thing. I reached over and slathered my creamy hand over him. I wasn't sure how my pussy would react to whipped cream, but at that moment I couldn't have given a flying fuck. His big whipped-cream puff came sliding down my canal. Every nerve inside of me was screaming with pre-orgasmic sensations. I swung my legs over his shoulders and screamed to my heart's content.

The whipped cream acted like a magic lubricant, making us slither together in a dream state. Soon pussy juice was added to the mix of whipped cream and sweat. The strawberries made their own contribution, oozing forth their prickly nectar. Radio Man and I were like giant babies, mushing around in our own gooiness. The outpouring of sexual energy made me erupt in a succession of repeated orgasms that was like a series of fabulous cherry jubilees. We were red, we were juicy, we were oozing sex from every pore.

I had one moment of clarity in the middle all this. I thought: So this is what it's like to be fully ripe.

I must say it was the best damn cake I ever had.

And hardly any calories!

UNDER-THE-TABLE MANNERS FOR MEN

Tired of the same old boring Friday night din-din at home? Table manners got you down? Then get down there with your table manners! Demand that your lover forget about his fork and knife. Ask him to lick sweet potatoes from between your thighs. Encourage him to butter your tits and lick, baby, lick! Emily Post will spin with envy! (Make him do clean up duty after you're completely spent.)

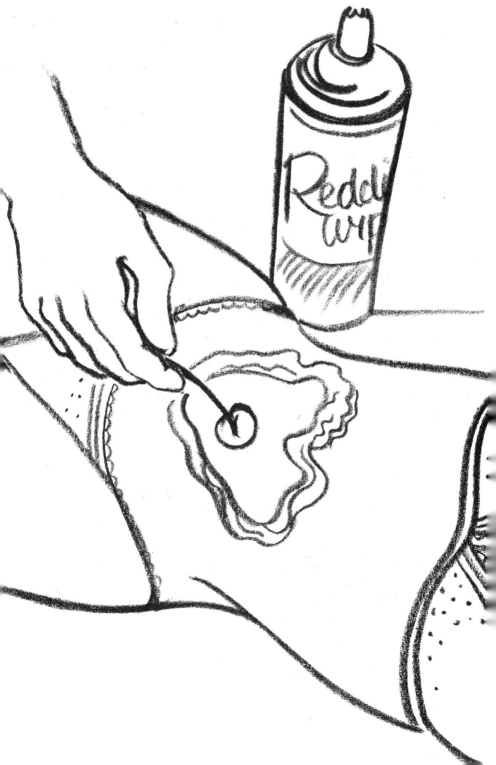

WHIPPED CREAM

First make sure the room is a warm temperature. Cover your bed, or a flat surface where you want to play, either with plastic or a sheet or towel. Plastic allows you to slide around more. Use something that you can comfortably mess up.

Have a large bowl handy. Fill it to the top with whipped cream. Whip well so that it reaches a fairly stiff, delectable froth.

Light candles.

Put on some music that inspires your groin.

Take off your clothes.

Take off your partner's clothes.

Start by sliding a fingertip through a mound of the whipped cream. Circle your partner's nipple with it. Be slow in painting your partner. Luxuriate in the sensation of feeling how the creaminess interacts with your partner's skin. Notice how it slows down your fingertips and speeds them up at the same time.

Tip your own nipples with the cream and dip them in his mouth.

Dig your hand in and scoop a large mound of whipped cream. Paint your lover's cock with it. Rub it all over his balls, particularly underneath. Stare directly into his eyes as you are doing it. Make sure you are on your knees between his legs so the visual drives him crazy.

Then put your tongue into action. Start at the base of his cock and start to lick him into a confectionery delight. Take each ball and suckle it to your heart's delight. (This is also known as "teabagging"—everyone's got food on the brain!) Use your tongue to draw a path all the way up to the tip of his penis. Slide your tongue into the little crevice. Do this several times to drive him crazy. Need I tell you more?

HOW TO HAVE FUN ON THE HOLIDAYS

Don't feel you have to confine yourself to birthdays.
There are holidays all year long for you to indulge your
food fantasies.

Easter Bunny

*Here's a no-brainer. Plant Easter eggs at the doorway, lead-
ing all the way to the bedroom. Whispering a little hosanna
to Hugh Hefner, put on your best Playboy bunny outfit.
(Don't forget the tail and white stilettos.) Bring a bag of
washed carrots. You can use a carrot on him, or he can use
it on you. Remember, carrots are good for your health. Bend
over the bed and let your man have his way with you.*

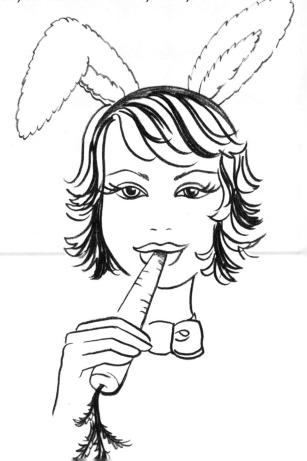

Fourth of July

Go ahead, celebrate your country. Where else do you have the freedom to express your sexuality, whatever it is, with so many like-minded individuals? Get a red, white, or blue G-string. Ditto for some matching pasties. Put on an Uncle Sam party hat and some outrageous false eyelashes. When the fireworks go off, light the sparklers in your hands, hat, and anywhere else you can stick them. (Go ahead, find a way.) Then deep throat your lover and wish him one hell of a Fourth of July. When he asks you, "Honey, why did you do this?" just reply, "I did it for my country, darling."

Christmas Elf

Have your man meet you for lunch at your home one wintry afternoon. As he makes his way to you through the cold, ready yourself by putting on a furry Santa hat, bright red lipstick, lots of eye shadow, a red satin slip dress, no underwear, and six-inch red patent-leather hooker shoes. Don't forget to have a manicure and pedicure in Christmas red. Leave the door open an inch, so when your man arrives he has to let himself in. As he stamps off the snow, you should be standing down the hallway a bit, legs splayed with a maraschino cherry in your mouth. Invite him into the kitchen for some hot fudge and ice cream—alternating hot and cold unexpectedly can be very sexy. How you heat up your man from there is up to you, darling.

SPICE UP A MEAL

- *Cook dinner naked, but for a pair of sleek stilettos.*

- *After dinner, lie back on the table, and present your dessert. Spread your legs and show your pastry.*

- *Après mealtime, suck a popsicle in front of your man. Slowly.*

- *There is nothing like a good can of whipped cream— everywhere.*

- *Fruit in the pussy is a good thing. For dessert, I mean.*

- *Dip your nipples in chocolate sauce.*

- *Sip your wine and then transfer it into his mouth.*

- *Dip his cock in a jar of chocolate sauce and enjoy your personal Yule log, ladies. (Gentlemen, try this yourself as a special treat to your lady friend during Christmas. I guarantee she will be very happy with Santa this year.)*

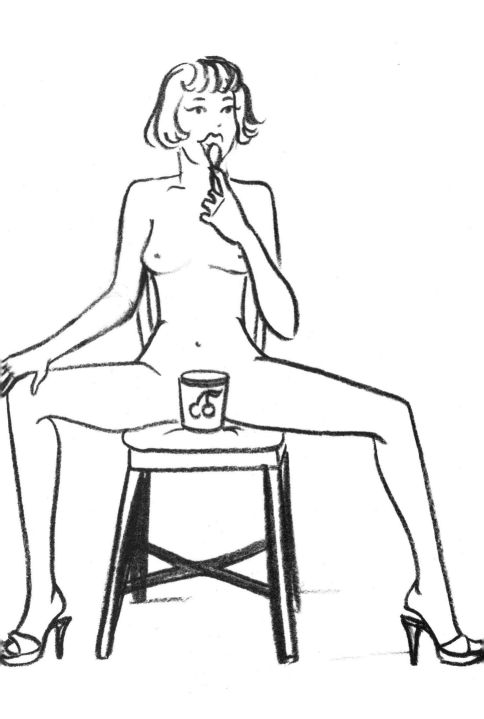

HOW TO TURN AN ORDINARY KITCHEN INTO SOMETHING MISCHIEVOUS

Use the following utensils in any way you desire:

- *Rubber spatula*
- *Wooden spoon*
- *Big metal spoon*
- *Cleaning brush*
- *Wool soap pads*
- *Small cutting board with a handle*
- *Wet dishrag*
- *Broom*
- *Feather duster*
- *Wire egg beater*
- *Cake server*

Use the following foods in any way you desire:

- *Cold or hot spaghetti*
- *Frosting*
- *Honey*
- *Ice cream*
- *Chocolate, strawberry, or pineapple sauce*
- *Cream or milk*
- *Strawberries, kiwi, pineapple, blueberries, citrus, watermelon, or bananas*
- *Ice cubes*
- *Whipped cream*
- *Cake, cannoli, or éclairs*
- *Cream-filled donuts*
- *Cucumbers, zucchinis, or carrots*
- *Breadsticks*
- *Anything else that resembles a cock, for God's sake!*

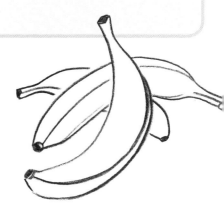

THE SEXIEST DINNER YOU'LL EVER HAVE
(Have your partner read this!)

Make a dinner reservation at a sumptuous restaurant. Tell your lady to wear the sexiest dress she owns but to wear nothing underneath. Nothing! Make sure you are dressed elegantly yourself. When you pick her up be sure she sees you survey her body slowly in front of her. Be obvious but don't be obvious, if you know what I mean. Present her with a bunch of the most exotic flowers you can find, something besides roses— fragrant orchids, perhaps. Kiss her and make sure you use your tongue. You want to get her in the mood.

Try to get a seat in a corner banquet so that you are sitting side by side. Touch her lightly from time to time; stroke her arm or run your palm down her thigh. While she is explaining her dinner preferences to the waiter, surreptitiously slide your hand between her legs and feel the warmth of her pussy. Order a lovely wine. Take a sip and then kiss her and drop the wine into her mouth. Cut up a piece of your dinner slowly, drag it sensuously across your plate, and offer it to her mouth. Follow this with a deep kiss here and there throughout the meal.

Dessert will come naturally.

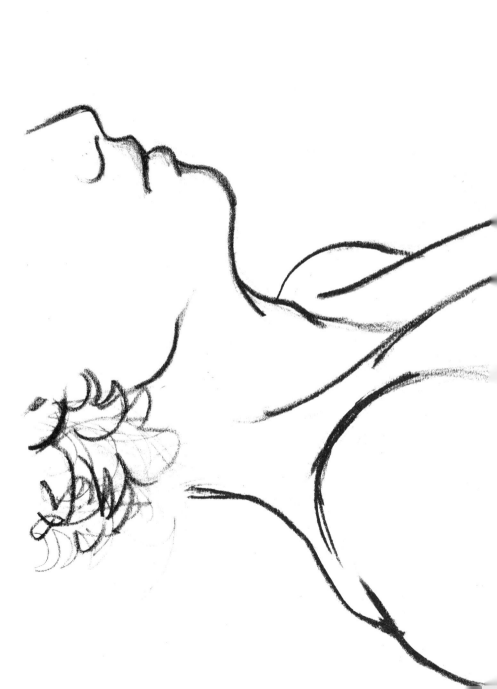

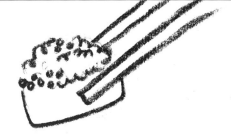

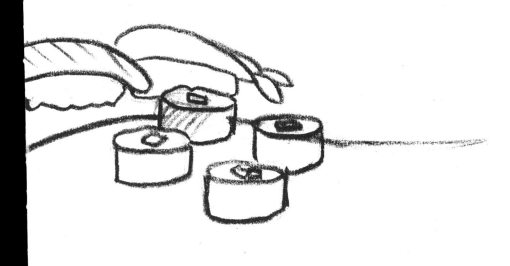

PUSHING THE ENVELOPE

Serve a meal on someone's body—yours, your lover's, or, if you're adventurous, a friend's body, creating a dining room table that lives and breathes (and moans). Just put everything right on that beautiful skin. You may want to tie his or her wrists and ankles to the table so the squirming can be kept to a minimum. Sushi is the "traditional" cuisine for this kind of service. Make it a real dinner party, if you dare. Anything goes here—just go with it, baby!

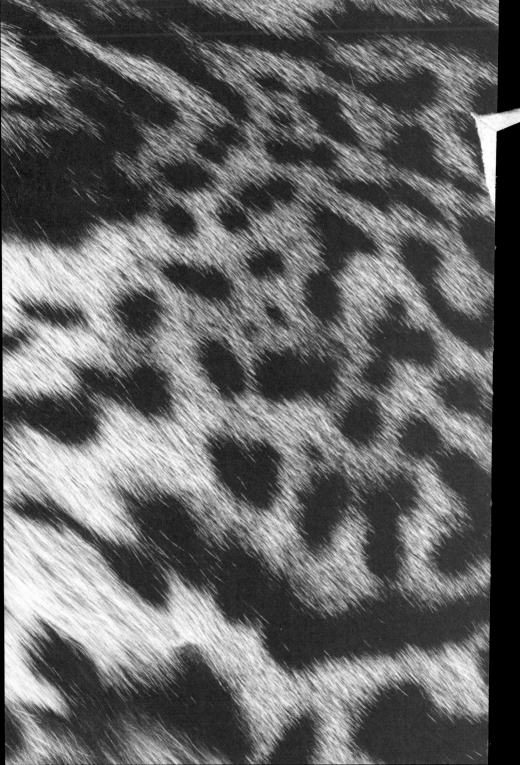

Of Human
Bondage

Tie me up! Tie me down! That movie didn't know the half of it.

Bondage can be one of the most creative aspects of a mischievous sex life—liberating for the person being restrained, and wild for the person doing the restraining. But it helps to know what you're doing.

You don't have to go to the extreme lengths I did to learn, since you mostly want to do this in the privacy of your bedroom, right? *(Right!?)* But since I was doing it professionally, I wanted to train with the best. I'd heard of the famous fetish diva Midori ever since I had first become acquainted with the Scene. Author of the book *The Seductive Art of Japanese Bondage*, she was raised a feminist intellectual in a Tokyo household and had enlisted as a U.S. Army Reserves Intelligence officer before becoming a well-known dominatrix out of San Francisco. She introduced the particularly lovely tortoiseshell body harness to the Scene and is amazing with numerous bondage techniques. When I got word that she was coming to the Fetish Flea Market, a biannual event held in Boston, I e-mailed to ask if she would consent to give me a personal training session. Thrillingly, she said yes.

〰〰〰〰〰〰〰〰〰〰〰〰〰〰〰〰〰〰〰〰

ILONA PARIS ON THE ART OF PLAYING

Remember when you were little, and it was so much fun to play doctor or cowboys and Indians? This is the same idea, but for adults. That is why we call it "play" in the Scene.

Using such components as fear and humiliation while playing will take you a long way. Think back to being a little kid, and the hours you would spend exploring each other's bodies without your parents watching. You used the guise of playing doctor, but it was an early exploration into erotic play, discovery, and titillation. Using your imagination is such an important part of play.

Picasso was a great believer in keeping your inner child alive in how you interact with your current world. People forget to do this as they mature. Be that child and play. Sexual mischief is all about play. When you use this concept of childish play and exploration, there is no need for shame. Instead, enjoy letting your inner self go and be free. The only limits are your own. Set them and be clear that they can always be changed as you go along.

〰〰〰〰〰〰〰〰〰〰〰〰〰〰〰〰〰〰〰〰

It turned out that she was staying at a Holiday Inn in Brookline right down the street from where I lived. I met her in the lobby. She was teeny for such a vicious diva, maybe all of five feet tall. She wore a black cashmere turtleneck, a black leather pencil skirt, and Calvin Klein spectacles. We jumped into my car and sped off for a training session in my dungeon.

Midori proceeded to explore my apartment and dungeon. She gave me ideas for everything. She looked at my 850-pound cage and suggested I use it for suspension. This would turn into a favorite with some of my clients. She surveyed my whipping wall and gave me ideas to make it more comfortable and safe. She suggested locations for hooks, and what sorts of handcuffs or rope bondage to use on a person's wrists. She came up with this crazy idea of cutting a large hole in the center of the wall so a person's face and head could go through it when I was torturing him or her.

THE WHY AND WHEREFORE OF HUMILIATION

Psychologists speculate that there seems to be something deeply cathartic about being humiliated to a point of powerlessness in front of another human being. The presence of another person makes the humiliation more intense and immediate, acutely increasing awareness and physical sensitivity. Jungian author Lyn Cowan states that it allows one to let go of old worn-out self images and attitudes, knocking down the outmoded boundaries and thereby freeing one to become more fully oneself.

Humiliation is akin to a live wire: Dare to touch it and you have no idea what it will shock you into. Most likely it will be self-discovery. There is no doubt that you will have to wrangle with your inner fears, but that is the core of what sexual mischief is about, my friends. It can allow you to evolve to the next place you want to go in life.

Her expert help on bondage took me farther down the path of S&M. What she couldn't help me with was the inevitable attraction I might feel toward a client. Here's the thing to keep in mind. You want to maintain the upper hand. You don't want to tip your hand by showing how much you're lusting after him. It is important that you stay in dominant mode, even if it's just for an hour or two. Trust me, it's hot.

Here's how I handled it with particularly attractive clients that I was ethically and legally prevented from lusting after. (Surprised to learn about my restraint? Here's something you may not know about me: I am impeccably ethical both as a Domme and as a therapist. Both roles require me to stay sexually neutral about my clients, and I am meticulously strict about not crossing that line. Getting sexually involved with clients is a no-no in both businesses, and I simply do not allow myself to play around with that divide. Interesting, huh? Because I was dealing with fire working both careers, it was mandatory to keep clear boundaries. I didn't want to end up as a newspaper headline, with *Entertainment Tonight* having a field day at my expense. And believe me, I was sometimes severely tested in this arena. It was all I could do to keep my tongue in my mouth.)

> "We can fight for equality during the day and at night get off on being tied up. It's not a contradiction. We've got to give ourselves permission to enjoy our fantasies."
>
> —Gabriele Hoff, Psy.D.

Robert was an environmental engineer and one of my favorite clients because of his streamlined, chiseled body. He was about forty and the ultimate yuppie. He was five-foot-eleven with freshly shaved, creamy white skin and brown hair well-trimmed and parted on the side. He had been a client of Midori's, which made me partial to him from the start—nor did it hurt (no

CLINICALLY SPEAKING

Though I am ethically and legally not at liberty to discuss my therapy sessions, I can relate to you some common observations and recommendations that I have consistently come across in working with counseling people in the Scene:

○ *Always strive to be up-front and honest with your partner.*

○ *Leading a secret life is guaranteed to bring strife into your relationship.*

○ *Never call your partner "sick" for his or her interest in kink.*

○ *There are many books on S&M, which you can read together in the privacy of your home.*

○ *A good way to start is to explore kink venues together, such as a fetish fair, leather society meeting, or S&M training class.*

○ *Talk together about what interests you. Don't scrunch up your nose in disdain.*

○ *Go to a sex store and buy some new items outside your comfort range.*

○ *Light candles, put on great music, and try out something new.*

pun intended) that he freely admitted he was a total pain slut. He always wore an expensive, crisp, white shirt with a Hermès tie, a look that is a complete turn-on for me. There is something about an upstanding man who is both "office attractive" and a pig that is just lovely to me. Robert was like a silken crème brûlée—wonderful to behold, with the smoothest abdomen I had ever seen. And then there was the cock. It *always* stood at attention. I found him utterly delicious.

It was rare to see such perfection in a human figure, and every time I saw it, I was able to admire it in a purely academic sense. The lines! The contours! He was a Donatello or Rodin, Robert was, made out of Carerra marble. With a cock equally hard. Banish those thoughts!

"There is a real voluptuousness in exposing oneself in weaknesses to the entire world."
—*Theodor Reik*

I walked into my dungeon to see him in the standard position, waiting for me on his knees before my throne.

"Stand up, slave," I said.

He stood with his hands clasped behind his back and his head bowed to me. This was a good slave who knew the etiquette. It always made it so much more fun when someone followed these commands to a T. I slinked over to my rope basket and chose a fifty-foot length of synthetic pure white rope. Let's just say I was inspired by that white shirt of his.

To make his reacquaintance, I came close, only a breath away from his face. I knew how the proximity of my physical being drove this man crazy. I looked directly into his eyes, like making eye contact with an animal to indicate your dominance. I kicked open his legs and commanded him to spread them. I applied some lube to an anal vibrator I held in my hand, and slid it smoothly into his asshole. Without blinking once, I just kept staring directly into those baby blues. I wanted him to know who had the power. He let out a small gurgle, and his head tugged backwards. The corner of my mouth twitched into a Mona Lisa smile. This was the effect I wanted. This was my power, my stand. He was mine, and I was perfectly clear about it. He would know, too, by the time I was done with him.

The vibrator would be held in place by the bondage I was about to perform—a tortoiseshell harness, I decided. I located the midpoint in the rope and draped it over his head so the midpoint hung loosely down to his stomach. Then I eased the rope over his shoulders and down his back, through his legs, and on either side of his balls. Some of the more elaborate bondage techniques require special care, which is a good thing in a session. The care I bring to the task always assures the client that I am paying close attention. I brought both ends of the rope up the front and draped it behind and over the loop pointing towards the stomach, then went back down between his legs and up the crack of his ass. Looping it from the rope around his neck, I made my way down and around to the breastplate area, hitching through the rope on the front and pulling sideways, almost as if I were crocheting. I pulled tight but made sure it wouldn't chafe the skin. You want the rope to be secure, but you don't want to stop circulation. (See Midori's *The Seductive Art of Japanese Bondage* for exact instruction.)

Remember that the point of all these S&M games (besides the heightened sexual titillation, *bien sur!*) is to lead to liberation and self-revelation. It becomes unhealthy and even pathological when it does the opposite and blocks self-knowledge.

I worked my way down his torso and then down his legs so he was wrapped up like a moth who had had an encounter with a spider. I pushed him back into my cage as he did his best to hobble backward. There was that impertinent cock of his, sticking straight out at me. I slapped it hard for good measure.

"Please Mistress, I just want to eat your pussy."

"You arrogant slut!" Again, I slapped his cock—*hard*.

It got harder.

BE PROFESSIONAL AT HOME: CLEAN EVERYTHING

If you are going to participate in S&M you need to be professional about cleaning things. Nylon rope is easy enough to clean. If you're just tying someone's wrists, you can spray the rope afterwards with Lysol disinfectant spray. If you have been doing more mischief, throw it in the washing machine on the warm setting with some good soap. But for other items such as gags, paddles, clothespins, and dildos, you must remember to disinfect everything. Clean dildos, vibrators and other equipment with hydrogen peroxide, or bleach wipes and disinfectant spray. Keeping everything clean is crucial for anyone who wants to engage in this sort of play. It's one aspect of keeping the play safe.

"Just sit on my face," he pleaded.

Normally a client doesn't speak this way to a Mistress. Nor would I allow it. But this guy was just too damn cute. I must say, this was one time when it was difficult for me to resist. I confess I felt my own moisture seeping through. And then I thought, wait a minute, this man has a wife. I have a career. No way in hell.

But God, it would be good.

I grabbed his left areola and twisted it as hard as I could. His head flew back from the pain.

"That is my answer, slut."

"Please, Mistress, one little taste . . ."

I took a deep breath and refocused myself. This was challenging but, I had to admit, fun (grin). I had to do something fast to shut his mouth before the temptation grew too strong. I grabbed a black ball gag and shoved it in his mouth.

"This is all I'm shoving in your mouth, slut."

All right, where was I? I chose some more white rope from my basket. Bondage is such a beautiful art form when you see the rope cleanly wrapped around and around, each loop perfectly in line with the next. I tied Robert's wrists to either side of the cage and then looped the rope through the harness on both sides so that he was now caught like an insect in the web I had woven, with the vibrator held into his butt hole by the rope harness. I stood back, crossed my arms, and murmured to myself, *Ahhh, Mistress is ready for her dinner*. I felt like nothing so much as the Wicked Bitch of the West. I'll get you, my pretty . . .

YOUR INNER BITCH

Being a bitch has gotten a bum rap. Try it yourself and liberate your inner bitch. See what you can do when you have another human being totally at your disposal. When he's restrained and can't lift a finger to stop you, see just how wicked you can be. Play the part! Be mean, be cruel, and give your victim the greatest thrill of his life.

I decided I wanted to go classical today and utilize basic black and white: white rope, black leather. I handled a soft black leather and fur eye mask, inhaling the heady smell of the leather deeply.

Jesus, I was in a state. Sweat was starting to pour between

my breasts underneath my latex. The only way to deal with this impudent sexy creature was to brutalize him. He was going to suffer for making me hot.

REMOTELY INTERESTING

Remote control devices are particularly sneaky. You can use them anywhere, and the surprise factor is worth its weight in gold. My personal favorite is a little silver vibrator inside a nude plastic penis with a remote control that you can operate from up to twenty feet away. It is small enough to fit into a vagina or anus, so place it in your favorite crevice and let the fun begin. (You may need to hold it in place with a tight pair of underwear, or if that's uncomfortable, I suggest panties that come with their own vibrator. These can be worn by men or women and pack a hell of a wallop.) The remote comes in the shape of a little box, which you can fit in your hand, purse, or pocket.

Go out to dinner at your favorite restaurant. Excuse yourself and make your way to the ladies' room or hat check area, or somewhere you can keep an eye on your playmate. Pretend to fish around in your purse while you discreetly turn on the vibrator. Watch your lover's face turn bright red just as the waiter is asking if he'd like another drink. Talk about your public displays of affection! It doesn't get more mischievous than this. Or go to the movies and enhance your movie viewing with your partner. I'd be careful of flying popcorn, though.

I waltzed across the room to where my remote control for the anal vibrator was located. I turned it on and watched Robert jerk to attention.

"Oh, is it working?" I asked innocently. I batted my false eyelashes delicately, and immediately strapped the blindfold on him, plunging him into darkness. My goals were twofold: to have him lose all bearings as to where he was and how long he would be there, and to enable him to concentrate solely on the physical sensations to come.

I buzzed him again. His face turned red, his ass cheeks twitched. His whole body squirmed as he moaned around the ball gag. This had to be the best job in town.

WHEELIES, ANYONE?

A fun item that is a good beginner's tool is the Wartenberg wheel. It looks evil to someone starting out, but can be pretty mild depending on how you use it. Originally used by doctors to find out if a person could feel sensation, it has a metal handle attached to a one-inch-thick rotating wheel with needle-sharp steel teeth all around it. The little teeth can unnerve someone who is blindfolded and doesn't know what is going on. Such devices can be bought relatively cheaply online or at a fetish event. Like many toys, it can be used to tease and tickle without causing real pain if the user knows what she's doing. Of course, if she really knows what she's doing . . .

I buzzed it up high and smiled as he nearly leapt out of his skin. Dance for me, darling!

The poor man was like a bundle of nerves built around the vibration in his anus. With no visuals to guide him, he had no idea when the next buzz was going to erupt inside the most private cavity of his body. I could control his whole being just by raising and lowering the dial on my remote. This was better than a remote control Roomba that vacuums the carpet while you steer it from across the room. But I betcha those Roombas don't beg to come, do they?

"Pweez, pweez, mustuss," he begged around his gag ball. His cock was the color of my nail polish. It was in such a state that it was throbbing with his heartbeat.

I decided to go for some CBT (cock and ball torture). I strutted over to my Craftsman chest. I looked at the array of torture devices lying in a row, displaying themselves to me. He needed to suffer. He liked it, he wanted it, and by Christ I was going to give it to him. He was a self-professed pain slut. *Aha*—I had it. A dozen red plastic clothespins twinkled before my eyes. They were from the Dollar Store at the mall. I clipped them all over his ball sack in a pretty row. They were baby-sized but vicious. Behind the clothespins I hung two huge wooden clamps with rubber tips, right behind his balls. Each one was about a foot long. I checked in: "How does that feel?" while squeezing his nipple to demonstrate who was in charge. I smiled. He shook his head up and down to show it felt good.

Then I got out my Braun electric toothbrush, a wonderful little number I bought at CVS. I turned it on and held it by his ear to freak him out. I held his ball sack up and ran the whirling brush underneath, slowly working my way up under the cock. This is a very sensitive area, as I witnessed by the hard monument standing erect before me. "Achhhhh," he sputtered, despite the gag. His poor rock-hard penis started to drip profusely. I slapped it to let him know he was a bad boy. I directed my toothbrush slowly around the

CREATIVE BONDAGE

You don't have to confine yourself to rope. Here are some alternatives:

Plastic Wrap

Plastic wrap is fun because it's cheap, readily available, and doesn't have to be cleaned afterward—you just toss it away. Around the holidays it even comes in bright colors! Like many worthwhile endeavors, it takes some practice to become experienced at wrapping someone. You might begin by wrapping your partner's arms behind his or her back, or placing a folded towel between the legs so the knees and ankles don't knock against each other, and wrapping the legs up snug. The trick is to wrap loose enough so the plastic doesn't cut off circulation, and tight enough so it doesn't fall off. If you are wrapping other parts of the body, it can be fun to cut out certain parts so you can play with them: nipples, balls, and so on. Use medical scissors (with blunt edges) to avoid unwanted laceration. Always cut carefully no matter what. Don't wrap the head or neck area. Be aware that the body sweats under this stuff so keep the person hydrated, and check for numbness or joints rubbing together and getting sore.

Duct Tape

Big, fat duct tape is great to use. It is quick, cheap, and again, can just be thrown away afterwards. It also gives great visuals because it comes in mean red and evil black. You can tie someone's hands in a ball or simply put tape across his or her mouth for a kidnapping scene. Imagine ripping it off! You can use duct tape for anything, but be careful that you don't wrap it too tightly.

Rubber Bands

I once saw a Dom use rubber bands to perform bondage on a woman's toes. You could do fingers, too—just be aware of the circulation factor. Remember, rubber bands are used to castrate goats (really!). Don't leave it on the cock overnight!

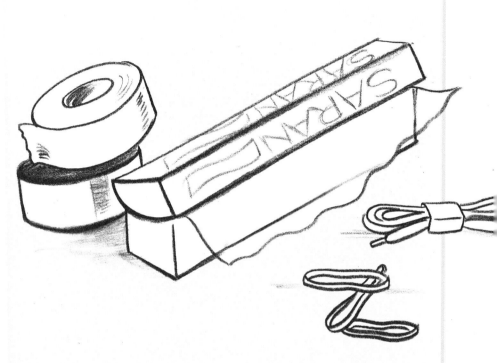

Shoelaces

Thick black shoelaces from men's construction boots are absolutely wonderful for tying up one's balls. Tie them around the jewels and then crisscross to lift and separate. Simply divine for tongue work if you are with your honey at home. Or you can just wrap the laces around and around the package. Get creative—cock bondage can be a lot of fun. See what you can come up with on your own. Clean the laces in warm, sudsy water. Keep a special pair to use only in sex play. You're worth it! (Besides, they only cost $1.29.)

rim and then over the little crack of his penis. His body spasmed as his cock flung upwards.

"You are nothing but an insect to me and don't you forget it." I flicked the little red clothespins still sitting at attention on his balls. He flinched.

I laughed out loud. God, I was feeling devilish. Things heated up quite a bit at this point, but my editor has insisted that I save those descriptions for my next book. Let's just say it involves a Wartenberg wheel and electricity.

Eventually it was time for a cool-down period. I always choreographed my sessions in three parts: First, warm up the client and ignite his tactile senses, then move into full throttle, and finally, finish with a cool-down and release.

If you're wielding the rope, you'll get high on ensnaring your partner and pulling him or her into your web. His eyes will become glazed with contentment (he'll become a "bondage baby") and he'll give himself up to you totally.

I removed Robert's gag and pulled off his blindfold, then waited a moment, giving him time to get his whereabouts. Next I undid the clamps and clothespins, suggesting he breathe deeply as they came off. (It hurts when the blood flows back into the skin.) Finally, I untied him.

Then I sat back in my red velvet throne, my latex gown glistening in the candlelight of my dungeon. It's hard work mistreating people. I think of all the naked men I've put under my spell and made crawl at my feet. Often I'll smile deviously, a sinful grin as I look down at the man at the base of my throne, naked on his back, legs spread-eagled to expose himself utterly to me. I cross my legs and press the toe of my red patent-leather stiletto into the base of his balls. Release? Sure, you can have your release at last. And tell me what a slut you are, darling . . .

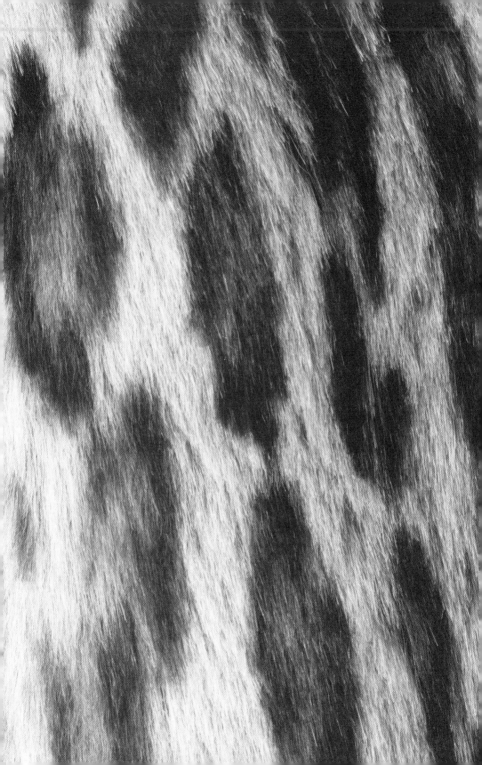

For The
Spanker
In You

Anticipation is all . . .

My research as a clinician has shown that one of the most important factors in S&M play is the anticipation of the act. People need and love those long, long moments of suspense—even if they last only a second or two. It's all in the timing. And nowhere is this more crucial than in the act of spanking.

But let me back up a bit, as it were, to a time in my life when I was in my deepest trouble. I came to the conclusion that I needed to clean up my act one day when I realized that flaming mini skirts with neon-yellow booties looked a bit tired when I went to church— ouch. Uh, not that I went to church much.

S&M isn't always about pain; sometimes it's about fear and control in a very subtle and wily way.

Sex was about the only thing that made me feel alive. I could fuck you till you screamed but the thought of sitting across the table from you and actually looking into your eyes and talking to you was something I couldn't even get my mind around.

SUSPENSE FACTOR
"Masochism has two characteristics:
the element of tension and the
tendency to prolong the suspense . . .
and the pleasure is more dependent
on this expectation of discomfort
than on discomfort itself." —*Theodor Reik*

It was time to take action. I joined Alcoholics Anonymous. Dutifully I listened to the drunkalogues and practiced my twelve steps. However, it did not escape my notice that AA might be a good place to meet men. In the early days of my sobriety, shopping for men in AA meetings was like walking into a candy store. There were tall, fat, thin, sugar-coated, cream-filled, and candied fruit. I had always loved candy.

One day I noticed a thin, forty-something man in AA with the craziest eyebrows I'd ever seen. I found them and him rather electrifying. It just so happened that he hung out with a friend of mine, who introduced him as Rupert, an indie filmmaker. "Do tell," I smiled, tapping my fingernails on the table. The three of us went for coffee, and Rupert mentioned that I should be a hand model because I have such beautiful hands. *Uh huh*. I'm sure he wasn't imagining my hands around his cock. As far as we were concerned, my friend didn't even exist at that moment. We had already entered the fuck zone, and both our minds were zinging. We agreed to meet for dinner the next night.

Anticipation, as they say, is all.

Rupert and I met 20 hours and 14 minutes later at a little bistro.

While we dined on fettucine al fredo, visions of fucking danced in our heads. He was a very funny man—always a plus. At 21 hours and 11 minutes, I confessed that I was fascinated by his stories of becoming a filmmaker. At 21 hours and 52 minutes, we were strolling around the city when we ended up—what do you know!—at my apartment. *Quelle surprise.*

He kept his cock a millimeter from my pussy for maybe ten seconds, but it felt like an eternity. By the end of those ten seconds I was so wild for it I was nearly salivating. When he finally put his cock inside me I was filled with delight. Longer . . . deeper . . . He was terrific. Those wild eyebrows of his were arched as he tossed me over onto my hands and knees. All of a sudden, just like that with no warning, he spanked my behind. Wow! This was new. It was 22 hours on the dot and I was learning something new. He spanked again. The combination of having to wait for his cock and then getting surprised by a spank was galvanizing, like hot and cold, no and yes. It seemed to punish me and reward me all at the same instant. Suddenly the little tips of my labia lips stood up to attention. Rupert continued to spank me until my ass was hot and tingling. Then he plunged his cock in my pussy anew, all the while continuing to spank me. This new dimension made the act more titillating than ever. Yes, I was a believer. Holy fuck!

It was probably because I was so open and vulnerable at this time of my life that I was receptive to being a spankette. So when I found myself back on top of my game again a couple of months later, what did I feel like doing, class?

That's right. Being a spanker.

When I was training to become a dominatrix I took several classes on spanking. I sat in a dusty loft at the New England

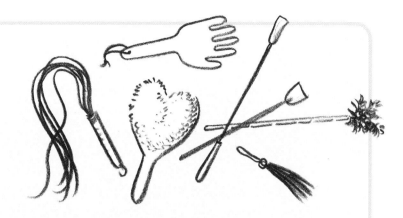

PLAYTIME: **TIPS FOR A GOOD SPANKING**

- *Make sure you have a naked ass to work on. (If you don't, there's another reason to punish it!)*

- *Spank around the area in different locations. You don't want to focus on one area over and over again.*

- *To find the sweet spot, locate the area right where you sit. This is the ischial tuberosity, the lowest bony part of the pelvis, sometimes called the "sitz bone" or "sitting bone." The meatiest part—that's where you want to smack.*

- *Change the intensity of the spank from soft to hard and back again.*

- *Use different implements to spank with. An old-fashioned wooden hairbrush is a classic for many, but you can use almost anything in the house!*

- *Build up to a nice red ass.*

- *A hand-shaped item leaves a nice imprint on the ass.*

- *You want to feel a certain amount of heat emanating from the skin, like lava from a volcano that hypnotizes you to jump in. Feel the heat, baby!*

Dungeon Society. Kinksters sat around on tattered sofas and banged-up bondage beds. There was a wall of chains to shackle people, a giant bird cage hanging from the ceiling, and a round medical bed in the corner, which could be rotated 360 degrees.

Mistress sat on a large throne. The naked submissive she had brought along for the demonstration lay across her lap—a favorite position for a spanking fetishist. He was a big man and his prominent belly hung over her legs. She demonstrated that you should spank around each buttock in a circular motion, never making the common mistake of hitting the same area repeatedly. She showed the location of "the sweet spot" for spanking, at the base of the buttock. While she spoke, the sub was quivering. Oh yeah, anticipation was definitely part of the scheme of things.

Mistress knew her topic inside and out.

After a while, everyone becomes quite particular as to whether they prefer to be spanked with a hairbrush, a bare hand, or something else. Play around to see which you and your partner like best. Maybe the kitchen spatula is his thing. Whatever you do, don't get stuck with one item. Stay open to various implements. Experimentation is the key.

I learned enough about the art of spanking to enhance my professional knowledge and craftsmanship. I had a spanking bench specially designed for me in LA—a nice little black leather and leopard-skin number. Before long I was proficient enough at the art of spanking that I could design an entire S&M session around it. Want to hear how one of those sessions went?

I had a client scheduled to arrive at 4 p.m. I was in full dominatrix garb: black lace-up boots with a dress made of silver chains held together by a few black leather strips. I was basically naked except for my black leather thong. I wore bright red lip gloss with sliver glitter in it and silver metallic eye shadow. I felt regal and ice-cold. No sooner had the church bells across the street begun chiming than the doorbell rang. (It always amused me how punctual S&M clients tended to be—they wanted to make sure they didn't waste a single moment!)

NOTES FROM THE PARIS REPORT

Spanking is a classic fetish. According to my research for the Paris Report, people tend to develop their fetishes early in life, mainly between the ages of six and nine years old. It is my observation that fetishes such as spanking, humiliation, begging, and anticipation are hardwired to the sexual stimulators in the nerve endings. Nevertheless, spanking enthusiasts in my counseling practice frequently have suffered (or enjoyed) a particular episode early in childhood that was deeply imprinted in their psyches during that time. Usually, a mother or an aunt might have spanked the child with a hairbrush or brought him into her bedroom and spanked him over her knee. These two scenarios seem to have powerful staying power—for males, and middle-class Caucasian males in particular. I believe they like being spanked because it reminds them of a maternal sentiment that made them feel cared for. They may have been getting spanked, but it proved they were worthy of the attention!

SPANKING GOOD ROLE PLAY

Role play is an important factor for the spanking fetishist. Many people like to recreate a spanking scene from childhood. Try the following scenes and outfits:

° *Dress up like a sexy schoolmarm with your hair in a bun and glasses. Be the strict disciplinarian with a ruler to rap his knuckles and anywhere else you see fit. Have him polish an apple for you and try any way he can to be teacher's pet.*

° *Play the sexy housewife with a blowsy housedress, loosely unbuttoned. Smile mischievously at your victim while kneading warm dough with both your hands (squish, squish). Slap his face with flour on your hands and tell him to behave.*

° *While eating dinner, tell your sweetie he has been a very bad boy and make him go stand in the corner. Naked.*

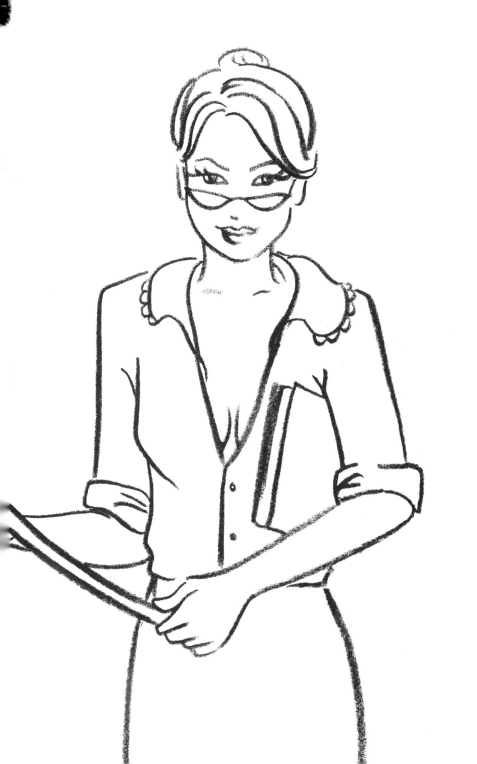

Now here was a specimen to behold. He was an Olympic rower with a stunning set of shoulders. Let's hear it for the Olympics. Truly, he looked like Adonis the Greek God of Rowing. But just to keep him from getting uppity I slapped him silly, collared him, and then attached a thin silver leash that matched my outfit. It gave me a kick to color-coordinate with my subs' torture devices. We made a nice pair, if I do say so.

"The love of a woman who sees the marks of nails on the private parts of her body, even though they are old and almost worn out, becomes again fresh and new." —*Kama Sutra*

I tugged his leash as he crawled down the hall, and I deposited him in my dungeon with instructions to strip and wait for me on his knees. Notice that there is a repetition to how these scenes are created. The submissive comes to expect and rely on this repetition for safety as well as for the excitement of the anticipation. My experience had shown me that making a person wait in this position, long enough for him to register the cool air on his aching joints, could spike up his anticipation level nicely. When I was feeling devious I'd sometimes have him kneel on some uncooked rice.

He was on his knees when I returned. I quickly kicked him in the derriere, grabbed his lush mass of his hair, and whispered "Are you ready for me?"

He tauntingly looked back and answered, "Yes, Mistress."

I gave him a good slap in the face just for his impertinence. His tanned body gleamed in the cool light.

He was a first-timer, so I had to strike a balance between his first-time fear and his desire for more, more, more. I applied leather cuffs to his ankles and wrists, fastened him to the spanking bench with chains, and locked him down with his derriere exposed.

People often like to be verbally humiliated while they are being spanked. Try insulting him while you spank and see whether that doesn't go straight to his cock.

Exposing the posterior always accelerates the sub's excitement, and I could see the desire in his flesh. He had two perfect pale cupcakes of a bottom. Not seeing any bony, weak spots or lesions that might get injured, I judged that he could tolerate a nice, moderate spanking. I slowly ran my hand over his buttocks, as if measuring him for a bathing suit, then gave him a quick slap. The sudden violence of it made him jump. I started to slap his two plump mounds; around and around the bum we go. It was fun for me to be able to do whatever I wanted, with no one to tell me *no*. Fun for him, too, obviously. *No* was the last thing on his mind.

He whispered, "I want to fuck you, Mistress."

I whirled around and slapped him. "You insolent slut, don't ever say that to me."

I took out a glove made of black rabbit fur, very soft and luscious, and ran it over his ass. Round and round I ran it over these twin mounds. He was warm to the touch and arched his

> Begging is also a component of S&M play.
> Making the subject or slave beg to be spanked not
> only puts him in a submissive position, where he
> wants to be, but it tends to prolong the process . . .
> upping that all-important anticipation factor.

backside up with pleasure to meet my touch. I smiled to myself.

"Oh, does the brat like this?"

"Yes, Mistress."

I wanted something to contrast with this sensation. Soft and hard, sharp and dull. The contrast between opposites counts for almost as much as the anticipation. Fortunately, these soft rabbit gloves had some nasty-looking steel claws attached to their tips. So in the middle of slowly rubbing the fur over his body, just when he thought he was getting a safe, sensual massage, I pulled out the claws and reminded him what he was here for. *Owwwwwwwwwch*—like a lowercase whimper of pain. No capital-letter "OUCH" just yet. I ran this deadly apparatus lightly over his backside—slowly increasing the pressure so that it left a trail of white marks up and down his epidermis. I had to feel my way along, getting into his skin, as it were, sensing when he was ready for the next step. I knew that if I proceeded too quickly I'd frighten him into self-consciousness. But if I went too slowly he wouldn't be getting his money's worth. He *wanted* to be frightened. Otherwise he'd be spending this hour at the gym.

I took out some wooden paddles, which produced a nice stinging effect. People seem to like either a stinging or thudding sensation. I started to paddle his buttocks, like a slow game of ping-pong.

Bam! Then faster: *Bam bam!* Then coming in for a smash shot. Whack! His cock flew up and he groaned.

RAISING THE ILONA FACTOR

Keeping your submissive in suspense is part of the game. Nothing ramps up the anticipation factor like having no idea, and no control over, what is about to happen. Try marching him into the bathroom and asking him to lean over. Then put on a pair of plastic gloves, spread those beautiful cheeks, and view his anus. (Always make sure the anus is clean when playing, folks.) Spray a dollop of shaving cream on your fingertips and apply it to the area. There usually isn't a lot of hair in this area, but it's all about the mind fuck. If you want to go further, hold the cheeks open and carefully shave the area. Can you imagine how freaked out and excited your playmate will be? You'll be the Cheshire Cat preparing Alice in Wonderland for the Queen of Hearts.

Wet a washcloth with warm water, wring it out, and gently wipe the anus. Stand back while holding the edge of the cloth and let it rip so it slaps his ass. Bull's-eye! It will have a wonderful stingy effect. And the visual will almost make you gasp. (Who says women don't get off on visuals as much as men?!) Imagine the tip of the facecloth snapping his sweet spot, then being slowly drawn along the length of his ass crack afterwards, up and down and up again . . .

"Someone likes this, I see."

"Yes, Mistress."

I gave him another smash, this time with a little topspin on it. Oh, that was good. Then a lob and then another smash, keeping him totally off guard, not knowing what devilishness I would serve up next. All the while I had to be careful, because I could mark him with this sort of toy, and it's generally not a good idea to leave evidence on the skin that wives or girlfriends might discover. However, many people like to have marks left on themselves. It is sort of like how strong you want your drink—your choice.

> Make him tell Mistress he has been bad and needs to be disciplined. Tell him to pick a number between 1 and 100, and have him count each time you spank him. They love this!

Locating a wooden hairbrush, I rubbed the prickly bristles over his behind, roughing up his skin even as I was soothing it. Whack! And whack again! Then I slid my hand over his rump to feel the heat. You have to learn to read the skin to make sure it's hot enough—the hotter the better. It's like putting your hand over a barbecue to see when the coals are ready. If you can hold your palm over the coals at a distance of ten inches for ten seconds, it's medium. If you can hold it for twenty seconds, the meat's still rare.

I judged this marvelous creation of mine to be well done. Just the effect I desired. I reached for a red plastic cane tipped with a hand-shaped paddle and started to pat his caboose, getting him used to the sensation. Every once in a while I delivered a nasty little slap with the hand part of the cane. Gradually I started to deliver the slaps closer together. In about two minutes I was whaling away, letting his sculpted cheeks have it from every angle. I could hear him whimpering but I showed no mercy. No back talk from him now! His cock was so eager it was dripping all over my spanking bench. I smacked him for this, then abruptly stopped and rubbed my hand slowly over the skin of his backside, which gave off a wonderful heat.

What came next? You'll just have to wait for the next chapter, dear reader.

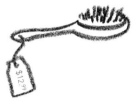

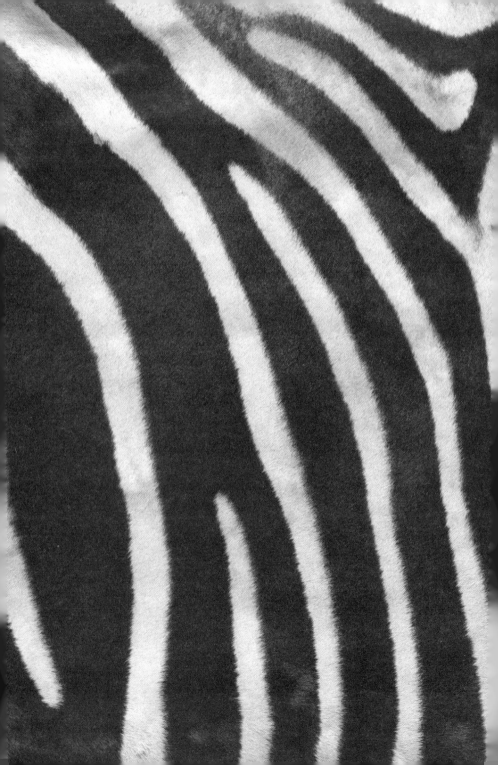

Whip It Good

*Don't let the word throw you.
It's not as scary as it sounds.*

Coolly I raised an eyebrow as I watched the Olympian Adonis crawl over the red carpet of my dungeon. What would I do for a closing finale? Aha, I had it. A little whipping on the whipping wall. This being his first time, I felt he needed a taste of everything. After all, trying S&M without trying whipping is like having a massage without the oil. It's okay, but why not add the extra dimension?

Yeah, I know how you probably feel. I was intimidated about whipping early on, too. I was first introduced to the art of the whip when I took a training course with Lady Stinger, a funny little Domme who had a weekly fetish club called LeatherUp. Every week I would drive my Beetle Shirley to her bungalow in a suburban subdivision (it never ceased to amaze me that these dungeons existed right in the heart of Middle America!) for lessons on everything from how to tie a corset to making a good bowl of chili.

The scene alone was worth the price of admission—she had a sissy maid named Mathilda who was at her beck and call round the clock. Mathilda dressed and worked as a male carpenter on his off hours, but on site he waltzed around in a frothy blue dress, lots of white petticoats, and a dirty-blonde wig à la Jean Harlow—with the added attraction of white bobby socks. Despite, or as a result of, being regularly used as a whipping boy/girl, Mathilda worked very hard to get his fingers into Lady Stinger's corset—a noble effort, given the fact that she was wearing a triple D. Another attraction was a frequent visitor, a middle-aged gent named Scottie who had a baby fetish and liked to be locked up in a giant cage with a coffee-filled bottle.

TIPS FOR WHIPPING

o *Practice, practice, practice.*

o *Train with the best whip Master or Mistress you can find.*

o *Make sure your feet are firmly planted when using a whip.*

o *If you need to wear glasses, for God's sake put the damn things on. This is not the time for vanity.*

o *Keep checking in with your slave to make sure he or she is all right.*

o *Never whip near the face or the kidneys, behind the knees, back of the arms, or neck. The upper thighs are okay; look for the meatiest areas.*

o *Practice, practice, practice.*

Lady Stinger's scene was primarily whipping. Whips were her specialty, her area of expertise, her raison d'être. I mean, this woman was Mistress of the Whip. It was rumored that her father was a lion trainer for a traveling circus back in Bavaria, and that he taught her how to use a bullwhip on kitchen chairs at the age of eight. She had been practicing for years and could do anything with a whip, even snatch a lit cigarette from Mathilda's lips at a distance of ten paces. Quick as a wink there'd be a snap and ashes flying around the room: the cigarette had been transferred from Mathilda's mouth to Stinger's. You wouldn't even see it coming. She also knew how to use a gun. But that's another story.

I was impressed, but mostly I was intimidated. The very sight of a whip threw a shiver down my spine. Of course, it was supposed to do that. It doesn't make that sinister *crack!* for nothing. One day I was watching Lady Stinger work on Stewart, another frequent visitor. Stewart was a commercial airline pilot who liked to wear a full latex bodysuit with a hood. He looked like the gent who was kept in a trunk in Quentin Tarantino's *Pulp Fiction*. He loved for Lady Stinger to whip him off and on for hours while he was dressed like this. Suddenly there was a whir in the air, and my behind felt like a queen hornet had attacked it. Yikes! Let's just say that Lady Stinger earned her name.

Lady Stinger broke me in by teaching me to do some light caning. Caning is done with a three-foot piece of bamboo of different widths (half an inch is nice). I had never caned anyone before in my life, and the first couple of times I felt like a fish out of water. I learned where to cane in order to maximize the chances of leaving marks, in case the slave wanted to take home a little souvenir. Submissives love, love, love to go home and look in the mirror at their marks. It is sort of like a badge of courage for them. I also learned how *not* to leave marks, in case someone at home would not be happy to find a classic "ladder" row of red marks up her partner's thighs and buttocks. Caning does not have to be hard to be effective. I've experienced being caned, and riding the pain of the cane is awesome—but when breaking in a beginner you want to go lightly until you have him hooked. Remember how in *The Da Vinci Code* some religious penitents would cane themselves to feel cleansed and renewed? It's sort of like that—it doesn't have to be really hard to get your point across. Once I had caning down, I began my lessons in flogging and whipping.

I practiced on a submissive man Lady Stinger had nicknamed Worm—a skinny little bald guy in his mid-sixties, wrinkled, crinkled, you might even say wizened; a devout believer in female supremacy, with thick black-rimmed glasses that looked like two television screens, and a thoroughly adorable smile. I used poor Worm's little behind like he was on a whipping post in medieval France. I mean, I can't believe I didn't wear it out. He loved every second of it, even begging me to shoot him in the butt with a blow dart.

BEING HURT VS. BEING INJURED

Lady Stinger impressed upon me how important it is to practice whipping. You need to know what you are doing. An injury is for keeps—you can't take it away after you hurt someone. To avoid injury with a whip, you need to concentrate with every ounce of your attention. There's a big difference between being hurt and being injured. Being hurt can be fun—lots of people derive sexual pleasure from pain. But being inadvertently injured is the opposite of fun. Receiving a whipping is a consensual activity; a person receives the pain—which ranges from the sensation of butterfly wings on the skin to the sting of a hornet— because he enjoys how it makes him feel. But accidentally snagging him in the eye because you don't know what you are doing is totally different and to be avoided at all costs.

Worm was Lady Stinger's tax accountant, and he was eventually to become mine as well. In fact, we made an arrangement whereby we agreed to swap specialties. He'd do the books for me, and I'd do the blow dart thing for him. (Most laymen assume that professional Dommes don't claim our earnings, but we want to stay on the up-and-up with the feds as much as anyone—so long as we have an accountant who understands the business.)

Balancing Two Careers

One time, my scrawny little sweetheart
of a naked CPA was spread-eagled on tiptoes to my
whipping wall, and I was dressed in my cat outfit,
shooting four-inch-long steel darts through
a giant tube into his shriveled little ass, when my
doorbell rang. I had gotten my schedules
mixed up and forgot I had an appointment with a
therapy patient. What was I supposed I do,
hand my patient a magazine and say, "Could you
just have a seat for a minute while I blow a
dart into my accountant's ass?" That was the first
and last time I mixed up my appointments.

Back to my Olympian rower, crawling in my dungeon, so excited with that big hard dick of his that it was more like scuttling . . .

I had changed into a full-length red Mistress gown, which swished around my ankles as I took long, dramatic strides in my red six-inch stilettos. I decided to warm him up with a little flogging. Floggers have a handle and usually many strands of leather, rubber, horsehair, or silk. They can inflict incredible pain or feel like a child's fingers on your skin. Flogging was quickly becoming a favorite of mine. I snapped on some Ibiza Summer Anthems—incredibly sexy music. I grabbed a red neon flogger made out of strands of rubber that looked like angel-hair pasta. I began swirling it around the rower's backside like a Kabuki artist putting on a show. I whirled it around in a circular motion so the tips brushed his buttocks, swirling and twirling.

Then I picked up two red suede floggers made of kangaroo leather, one in each hand. (This maneuver is referred to as "Florentine.") I slowly draped them over his back, letting them run the length of his skin. This was a wonderful way to sensually tease the skin for him and for me at this point. Sensual teasing paired with pain, whether gentle or harsh, is delightful. I swung the floggers as if I were a flying bird while I slowly moved one leg out in front of the other in an erotic dance of pain and sensuality, dancing and gyrating all at one time. This whole art is all about theater, don't forget. Mesmerize your slave, enticing him to come back for more, developing a hunger in him that only you can sate.

Again I had to judge how hard and fast to go. I took a moment to ask how the rower was faring.

"I'm fine, Mistress," he replied.

"Good, little slut. Keep me informed as to how this is feeling to you."

I swung a flogger up to caress the crack of his ass and under his balls, loving the way the muscles in his buttocks and back twitched each time. It was time to cool down this part of the choreography before moving on. I took out a leopard-skin paddle with rabbit fur on one side and painted his body with fur. He melted like butter.

I could tell he wanted to be whipped, but since this was his first time, we were going to go easy. Our little warm-up with the floggers taught him that he could trust me with the pain level. There wasn't going to be much pain, just a gentle stinging, like hail on a winter day hitting your face—but in this case it would be his behind. I took out a long yarnlike apparatus that I'd found in a pet store for my cat, Sushi. I stood at his side and lightly flicked it so it curled around his cock. This was fun and he loved it—although Sushi was wondering what the hell I was doing with her toy.

A CRACK BY ANY OTHER NAME

That fearsome and fulfilling thwack *is the result of the whip's tip (the "popper") traveling along the length of the whip faster than the speed of sound—at more than 700 miles per hour. It actually creates a vacuum in space, and since nature abhors such things (hell, I hate to vacuum, too), the air rushes back in with a popping sound. Your own personal mini sonic boom!*

I decided to position him against the wall, where he could feel the effect along the length of his backside. Standing him up, I attached his wrist and ankle cuffs to my whipping wall. What a sight. Once again I was struck by the vision of stunning muscle and flesh as if I were actually viewing a piece of sculpture from the Vatican. I had rarely seen a man this stunning. It had an effect on my central nervous system as well as between my legs.

I delicately traced my fingers along the sinewy trails of his backside, which seemed to be calling out to me. I wanted to torture and caress all at the same time. I started each movement at his sweet spot, traveled up his spine and across to the points of each shoulder, getting into the music and following the skin wherever it took me, creating a design of my own inspiration.

TYPES OF WHIPS

Bull whip: Catwoman, call your office! These are the super-long (six- to eight-foot) whips favored by Hollywood, with a wooden handle and rawhide core. Built for durability, they are among the most visually impressive, though they are not really the best for cracking.

Blacksnake whip: Similar to a bull whip except that the handle is more flexible, due to its being made of rawhide instead of wood. A matter of personal preference.

Signal whip (or singletail): Similar to the bulls and blacksnakes, but half the length (three to five feet), thus making them easier to crack. Better for indoor use.

My all-powerful motions with my bare hand seemed to electrify his nerve endings. At the same time I was picking up on something else he seemed to be radiating: fear.

"What are you afraid of?" I whispered in his ear.

"You, Mistress."

I let a moment pass.

"You should be," I snorted, grasping the woven purple and black leather knob of my singletail. Again, I knew that I wasn't going to inflict a lot of pain on this guy. But at this moment, expectancy was worth its weight in gold. I wanted to ramp his anxiety level up to the sky. I stood behind him in a firm stance. Biding my time, I focused on slowly unfurling my whip on each upper thigh and then on each side of his upper back. Ping, ping, ping. It reminded me of a snake unrolling its tongue.

The delight for the recipient is the anticipation before the sting. Softly, softly. Of course, the other end of the spectrum is to really let it rip and to actually slice into the skin. I never went there. Not only can this cause serious (as opposed to fun) pain to the client, it can also ruin the whip. Nothing destroys a nice set of threads faster than a few drops of blood. In general, you want to enthrall the skin—not exfoliate it. If the skin is reddening, that's nice. But you want to keep the blood well beneath the surface, not spurting through.

Sadomasochism challenges you to forge through inner blocks within yourself. By cracking yourself wide open to new potentialities, you can avail yourself of a heightened spiritual life, if you so desire.

I went for each shoulder, then each buttock in a crisscross motion. The effect is akin to soft kisses with a bit of a bite. It is amazing how a little pain results in an arousal of the sexual organs and in fact the entire nervous system. Wow, what a wonderful creation this human body was. I looked at this one before me with pleasure and curiosity. Why did he need this experience in his life? Why was he so evidently hardwired for it while others could care less? What role did I play in all this? My desire to teach others about pain's true nature never ceased to pique my own curiosity.

THE CARE AND HANDLING OF YOUR WHIP

o *Do not buy a whip at a fetish fair. Buy a whip from a Master whipmaker who makes exquisite pieces. (The best way to find him is through word of mouth, but you can also check out ads in the backs of reputable leather and fetish magazines, as well as on the Internet.)*

o *A whip should have a lead-shot handle and should be woven of sturdy leather.*

o *Try using a whip made out of a rope cord in the beginning if you are scared but curious. Then wet the cord if you want to kick it up a bit.*

o *Do not fold the whip. Hanging it by the handle will prolong its life.*

o *Do not drag your whip on the floor.*

o *Replace the tip when it is worn out. (Don't ask me how to do that; that's what slaves are for.)*

o *Avoid that sticky red substance known as blood.*

Always in my mind was the paramount question: How far should I go? Many people love the pain but many others love a gentle flutter awakening their skin. It's a delicate balance—the difference between a quiet "yow" and a giant "YEICH!" A pro Domme is expert in this balance, sensing her way along, but there's no reason why a layperson can't learn to maneuver just as well in the privacy of her own home.

I cracked the singletail in the air with all my might—a deafening *thwack* that scared the shit out of my slave, though it was nowhere near him. I tried not to giggle as my cat, Sushi, performed a maneuver similar to that of a Tazmanian devil. With a great show of kindness, I gently rested the palm of my hand on my Olympian's face. "Even more scared now, darling?" I asked innocently, petting his face.

I did this for about twenty minutes, alternately terrifying and then soothing him, switching back and forth between different styles of whipping. Finally I took a round paddle with leather on one side and shearling (the short wool from a yearling sheep) on the other and languidly massaged his skin with it. Notice how I frequently utilize something soft and sensual before or after a scene to reassure the individual that he or she is safe. When I felt he was sufficiently cooled down, I unsnapped the hooks of his cuffs. That way his hands were free to do what they were dying to do . . .

DON'T BE AFRAID TO LAUGH!

Let me tell you about my laugh. Sometimes it's liquid, and people say it's like a rippling fountain, warm and sensual. Sometimes it's zany and reeks of craziness. I like to really get into it like a balloon being released and flying into the sky. It's totally infectious when it's like that. People crack up. But my best laugh for S&M is a cruel laugh. It's a little bit scary. In fact, quite a bit scary. But it's so much fun to let loose with it.

I took out a spreader bar, put it between his legs, and ordered him into my steel cage, which was the size of a large phone booth. "Would you like a release?" I purred.

I thought his eyes were going to roll back in his head as he gasped, "Yes, Mistress."

I closed the door to the cage and locked it. I took my seat in my throne, slowly crossed my ankles, and tossed him a little white towel.

"Make sure you ask for permission before you come, slut."

I sat back to watch the show. Have you ever watched a man jerk off? I must have seen the performance a thousand times, but it never lost its power to captivate me. It was a miracle each and every time. How could a little rubber-necked clam like that turn into a fearsome sea monster? He looked a little like a school kid, proud and bashful both, as he surreptitiously spit in his hand to lube it, then slowly rubbed his cock. Gradually it grew to a rock-solid nine inches. Hot damn.

"Very nice," I stated. I felt it was important to give support. *Righhhht.*

Faster, faster, faster. He kept his eyes glued to my body. Who knew what was going on in that pea-sized male brain of his? Probably cunt cunt cunt. Kiss kiss kiss. Whip whip whip. I had to admire the single-mindedness of his drive.

"May I come, Mistress?"

"Let me think about it," I said. "Um, yes, you may come."

Right on cue, he was like a geyser shooting his spray. Ah, the wonderful power of hydraulics. He wiped his cock and smiled bashfully, like a third-grader who had just given the teacher a flower.

"That is your session." I smiled. I was always quiet at the end of a session. A lot had happened, and it was almost a moment of reverence. "*Namaste*," I said, bowing slightly. "The light in me salutes the light in you."

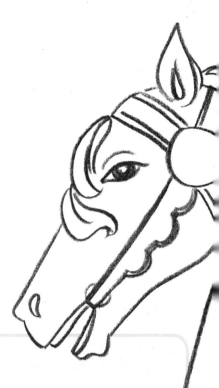

HOP ON THE MERRY-GO-ROUND

S&M is similar to walking through a looking glass into a wonderland of pain and pleasure, suffering and joy, on a merry-go-round of ecstasy. Once you can be open to admitting that you enjoy these elements together, you slide into a playground ripe for exploration and revelation. It is difficult for anyone to take this risk because in essence you are admitting you are pleasured by that which hurts you. The surprise of the revelation is that S&M has the potential to be a sublime experience in your life.

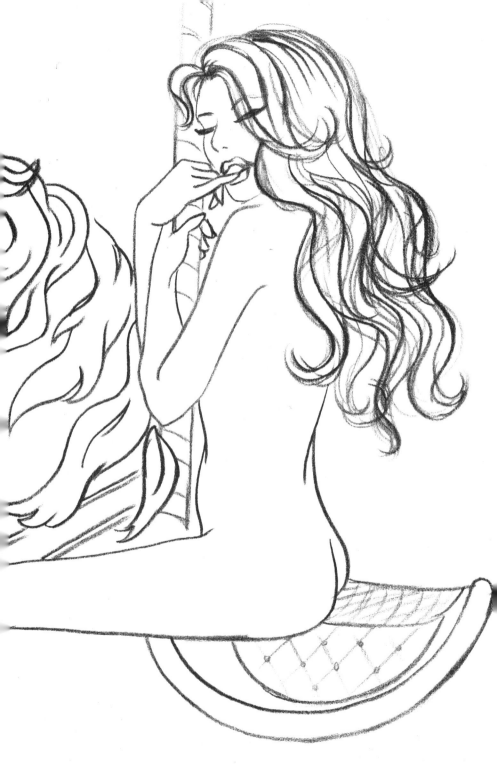

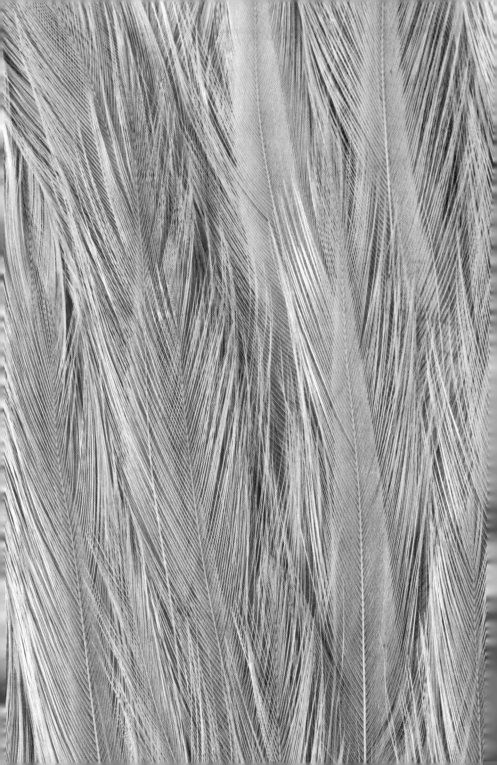

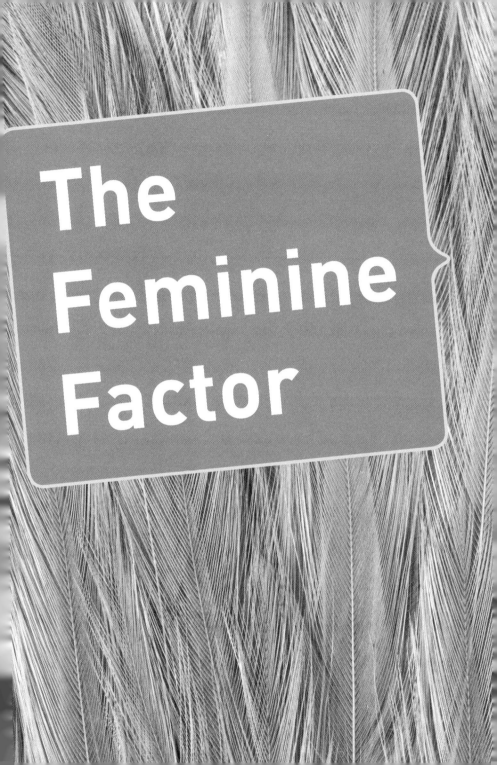

The
Feminine
Factor

Mango, anyone?

I love men. But when you're livin' in a Ben & Jerry's world, it's just too sad to limit yourself to only one flavor. So I had had some experience with women before I got a call from one for a session. But it was a surprise nonetheless.

It is highly unusual for a woman to call a dominatrix. In fact, it's so rare that some Dommes tend to give her a bargain rate or not charge her at all. I wasn't quite that lenient. I figured if I was going to go to the trouble of beating someone professionally, then I wanted top dollar.

Later that evening the doorbell rang, and I answered the door. A petite woman, about forty years old, stepped into my apartment. She looked like your average businesswoman, but with a hungry look in her eye. I was expecting someone severe because she had had a heavy accent on the phone, but she seemed demure, with dark hair and smoky brown eyes. I towered over her in my five-inch stilettos. She looked up at me and whispered, "Are you a woman?" I cracked up, then grabbed her by the neck like the leopard I was and slammed her against the wall. "Yes, I'm a woman. Are you afraid?" I peered into her face.

She trembled with fear and desire.

I commanded her to get on her hands and knees and follow me down the hallway into my dungeon. I instructed her to undress and wait for me naked in front of my throne. Her forehead was to be on the floor with her hands on either side of her head. I left the room for a few minutes to give her time to prepare herself.

I walked around my apartment for a few minutes to get myself psyched. She had balls, I had to give her that—coming over here by herself the way she had. I wondered what motivated a woman like her to seek out such an intense fantasy. And I felt an unusual little tingle somewhere deep in my psyche. The energy from knowing a woman was in my dungeon was distinctly different from knowing a man was back there. I ruminated on what I might do to torture this woman and also thought about what turned me on when I had been a submissive. Okay, ready or not, here I come, I said to myself.

Slowly I opened the door to my dungeon. There she was, a naked woman kneeling in homage. I was in my black latex number. Slowly I walked all the way around her and then grabbed her hair, pulling her into a standing position. I yanked her head back into the crook of my shoulder and looked into her eyes. It was clear she wanted this so badly. Her desire shone through, if I may wax poetic, like a beacon over a moonlit sea.

I could feel myself getting into a rhythm and

Alfred Kinsey's research in the 1950s indicated that the majority of people appear to be at least somewhat bisexual.

starting to become one with her. To be spiritually in sync while practicing S&M was a surprising experience. I stored this away in my brain for later observation. The power had arrived.

SEX SHOP ETIQUETTE

Many sex shops are more than a little sleazy and can make you feel awkward. My advice is to resist the discomfort and be as brazen as you can be. Stroll up and down the aisles with confidence. Bring your items to the front, look the cashier square in the eye and say, "Got any discounts if I buy in bulk?" (It does help to be a bit of an exhibitionist.)

If you can't quite pull that off, avail yourself of two other alternatives:

1. *More and more cities feature sex shops designed for and run by women. Softly lit and festive, they're like night and day from the sticky linoleum joints that are slowly being phased out. Support your sisters, sister!*

2. *Remember that the Internet is your friend. Shopping online for sex toys is almost as good as shoe shopping at Barneys. You'll love it!*

I released her and told her to stand still so I could inspect her. I ordered her to hold her arms above her head while I walked around her again. There is nothing like standing totally naked in front of someone while in a submissive mode and having every inch of your nakedness inspected and reviewed. It never fails to go directly to that little point at the tip of your clit or cock, which makes it feel immediately electrified. I slowly ran my hand down her back and over her derriere and murmured, "Very nice, slave, very nice." Her body was softer, more pliant, and more capable of being easily bruised than a man's. This made me feel both sympathetic and cruel, an exciting combination of feelings. I was very aware that there was no cock to play with.

PARIS REPORT CAPSULE

Sexuality can be quite open in the Scene, thus allowing for a variety of choices. Of the respondents to my survey (48 percent of whom were female), 50 percent were heterosexual, 23 percent were bisexual, and 11 percent called themselves ambisexual (or indiscriminately attracted to either sex).

I reached out and slid my fingertips around her nipples. Her breasts were ample with large protruding areolas the size of rosebuds. I twirled them in my fingertips and squeezed them until she winced in pain. Ah, that looked good. Let me do it again.

I selected a piece of poppy-red silky rope out of my rope basket and tied it around her breasts, sort of like a perverted Cross Your Heart bra except there was no bra—just a wonderful lifting and separating of her breasts. Red suited her features. *The better to torture you with, my dear.* Then I pushed her onto my bondage bed, designed so that my client's legs were spread apart to give me full access to her crucial anatomy. First I attached burgundy-red alligator mitts on each of her hands. They buckled at the wrists with a clip at the tip. I pulled out another burgundy-red rope and quickly went to work weaving a web that would ensnare my victim's body so she couldn't move. Clients always loved this—not only for the visual intricacy but also for the paralysis it provided them. Being tied

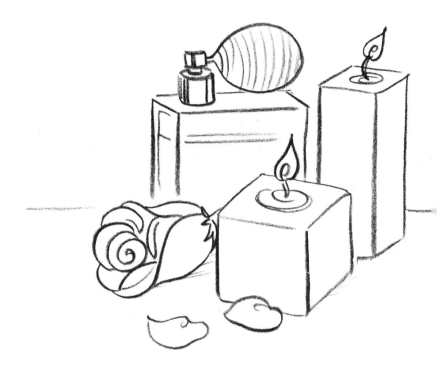

ILONA PARIS ON WOMEN

There's definitely a difference in making love with a woman. Their delicacy is similar to an orchid's. They are so much more responsive than men—you can see it in the way they arch their necks and moan in delight. Their fingertips are like sensitive jewels. Their smell is heady but sweet. Therefore you need to be clever in how you set your designs. If you're not going after a woman yourself, have your partner read this!

Foreplay

Women need foreplay. I find receiving photos of someone's cock or pussy boring and uninformative. A woman wants to know who you are and what makes you tick. She would rather have witty repartee than a Rembrandt of your cock. Seduce her with your eyes. Caress the back of her hand. Brush her hair off her face. Feed her food during a meal. Go for subtlety! Don't think of ramming or cramming . . . at least not until she's begging for it.

Little Gifts

Women love gifts: a bottle of perfume, bubble bath, lotion, flowers. Forget chocolates—too many women are watching their weight these days. Send cards that are creative. Women love to know that you are thinking with your mind and not just your sex. Romance, romance, romance—combined with an infusion of deviousness—is what will turn her on.

Do the Unexpected

Never underestimate the power of surprise. Blindfold your lover and bring her to the aquarium. Book a weekend at a spa for the both of you. If you can afford it, sweep her away to the Caribbean for the weekend. Don't just reserve dinner at the Four Seasons—book a room overnight. Go the extra mile and have candles, flowers, and petals all over the place before she arrives. (You'll be amazed how bellhops and other hotel personnel will get into this and come up with extras.) Have a beautiful, sexy piece of lingerie waiting for her on the bed. Fill the tub and give her a luxurious bath. Slowly and seductively massage every part of her body with a dripping loofah.

up and unable to move always allowed a person to think he or she wasn't responsible for whatever happened in a scene. *Yeah, right.*

I bent over and whispered in her ear, "Be still, my pretty, or I will have to hurt you."

I looked between her legs and smiled as I observed she was already wet. "You disgusting slut! You are itching for this, aren't you?" I slapped her inner thigh. Her labia were swollen and looked like a little penis. The outer lips were a deep purple, reminding me of one of Georgia O'Keeffe's New Mexico paintings.

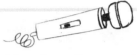

GOOD VIBRATIONS

Women respond well to anything that vibrates. The Hitachi Magic Wand vibrator is your specially intense friend. Little vibrators that you can attach to your fingertips are nothing short of divine. Watch your beauty melt before your eyes as you massage her body with these wonderful toys. But remember to build up to it. Start with a little pressure and continue to intensify it as you go along—slowly. If your partner knows how to swirl this toy around your clitoris, you may very well have something close to a religious experience. A similar apparatus is the vibrating glove—a black glove made of nylon, and each fingertip vibrates. Oh my!

I inspected my red tool chest filled with apparatus. *Hmm*, what would I do to this woman to thrill her even more? No matter how much preparation you do for a client, you have to stay open to the impulses of the moment and be able to improvise. Something about the way she lay there with her swollen labia reminded me of an earlier scene in which medical clamps had been put on my labia. Having your lips go numb from being clamped is surprisingly stimulating. It feels as if you have just been fucked by a squadron of hot marines. Yes, that was it! I pulled out a few clamps, and she watched, transfixed, as I skillfully attached them to a lip on each side. I then clipped some hot pink vibrating nipple clamps to her nipples. I turned them on low and stood back to see the effect this was having. Looking up at me from the bondage bed, my client was smoldering, her lower lip trembling. Her hands kept twitching, unable to do anything because they were helpless in the mitts. I laughed in her face but loved the feeling of strength that it gave me.

REALITY DILDO

There's no end to the variety of dildos out there—some subtle, some not. Your evil Mistress Ilona is wild about rubber dildos, which come in all sorts of colors and sizes. They're particularly comfortable on one's inner walls. Just remember to use plenty of lubricant.

I was inspired. I decided we were going to have a vibrating extravaganza. I took a silver vibrating egg, stuck it in her twat, and turned it on. *Take that, you little slut.* Then I stuck another one in for good measure. *Ha!* Even though they were on low, she started to squeal, squirming with pleasure. I knew that having a vibrator up your twat was an incredible experience—making you feel very alive but also very afraid that you're going to lose all control. It was wonderful to know that I could bring someone to such a state of ecstasy. I now knew how men felt when they were with a woman— whole, strong, and in charge.

It was time for the pièce de résistance—my Hitachi Magic Wand vibrator. This is the mother of all vibrators and guaranteed to send a woman to another planet. It has a big head and can be regulated from a kitten-like purr to a roaring cosmic vibration.

I stood between her legs and lovingly placed it on her clit. She started to yelp. That wasn't a good thing because of my nearby neighbors. I slapped a piece of duct tape over her mouth. Now that looked good. I slowly rolled the vibrator around her little pea pod, teasing the area like a pussy playing with a mouse. Gradually I rotated the dial until everything was turned on high. I moved the Hitachi around in different areas and varied the pressure. I continued with the circular motion. *Around and around you go, my dear.* Because I was a woman myself, I knew just when to pull back and let her catch her breath, bringing her to higher and higher levels of ecstatic anticipation.

Finally I could tell by the quivering inside her thighs that she was ready to come. I looked down at her body and asked, "Would you like to come for Mistress?"

She nodded her head vigorously. I had to laugh. It was gratifying to turn a woman on and do things to her that I knew felt really good.

The Hitachi and I struck gold.

Though it wasn't the first time I'd experienced the pleasures of the feminine factor, it was my first professional experience doing so—and it felt like quite an accomplishment!

Get a vibrator that plugs in—
electricity beats the energizer bunny every time!

FANTASY TIME

Men love to imagine two women together. Have you ever suggested to your partner that you might entertain that notion? Or walked him through it? How about three women? I had that very experience—described below. Feel free to use it for your own fantasy!

When I first moved to Boston, I became friends with a beautiful woman named Sabine. We worked together, and soon began going out for cocktails. We both loved dancing and dressing up in crazy matching outfits. We would go shopping in search of theme outfits that we could wear together. We loved going out to grab some cocktails and get toasted.

Sabine had a live-in girlfriend named Stella, a tough woman with short, bleached blonde hair. I started staying at their pad on weekends, and neither of them seemed to mind when I sometimes brought home boy toys for my enjoyment.

Sabine and I adored being big city girls in Boston. Everything seemed special and new. We had no idea what we didn't know. One night when Stella was out we decided to team up and troll for men. Separately, we figured, we were appealing enough, but together . . . well, any man that got us would have a lucky night.

Sabine and I went into action. After a few drinks at a bar one night, I found myself snooping on Danny, who was about five-foot-ten, with black curly hair, deep brown eyes, and a body like something out of a Calvin Klein ad. We picked that boy right up, the three of us dancing like fools. Danny asked if we wanted to go on his friend's boat. Sabine's eyes twinkled back with agreement. God damn right we wanted to go on that boat. We piled into her

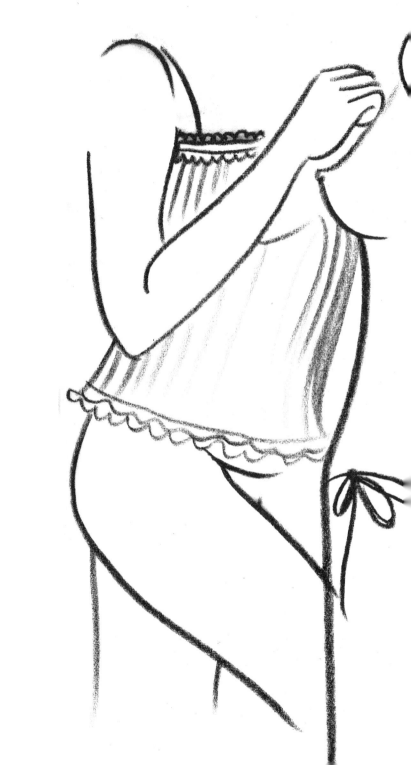

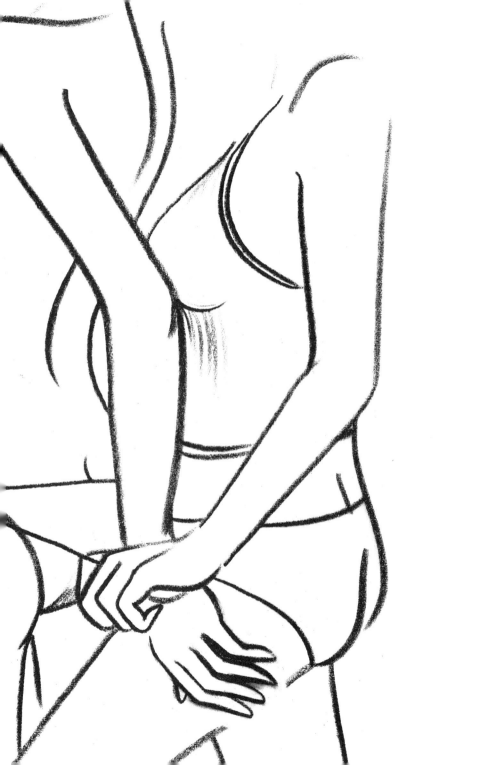

borrowed convertible and went down to the wharf to meet the "big boys," the people with real money. It turned out that Danny was on the crew of this 160-foot cruiser yacht. I had never seen anything like it before in my life—so elegant, with crystal chandeliers, a sculpted stairway, and a bar stocked with everything. We helped ourselves to some Veuve Cliquot, then flung our glasses over the side—a must for everyone on a 160-foot yacht—and proceeded down the hall to the master bedroom.

I lay down in the middle of the bed, which by itself was the size of a boat. Danny thought this was a wonderful idea and jumped on board as well. Then we both looked at Sabine, but she was not happy with the setup and made it known that she wanted to leave. What a party pooper. Danny declared that he wanted to come with us, but we ordered him to freshen up our drinks first. While he was off doing this, we decided to jump ship—literally. Try jumping to a dock in four-inch heels. Sabine sprained her ankle so badly we thought she'd broken it.

By the time we'd hobbled back to her apartment, I was feeling very woozy from all the mixed drinks and champagne. Usually when I feel woozy I feel horny, and it was no different this time. I thought to myself, "Well, I haven't had much luck with men tonight. Why don't I try something different?" Luckily Stella was home, and she and I soon found ourselves snuggled together on a loveseat as Sabine used the bathroom. I remember looking at Stella's soft pink lips as though I had never seen them before. Suddenly they appeared good enough to eat. I had never kissed a woman, and when we started to make out it was like brushing my lips across fine silk pajamas.

Sabine emerged in a diaphanous white gauze gown with her Rapunzel-like black hair flowing down her back. Stella and I both raised an eyebrow at each other. Clearly she was teasing us to attack her. We got up, led her into the bedroom, and threw her onto the bed where we both smothered her with kisses. Sabine lay back with her raven hair spread out over the pillow. She had the most marvelous smile on her face as we ravaged her. She closed her eyes in delight, and we moved down from her neck to her clavicle, then to her breasts. We each took one breast in our mouths. First I bit her brown areola. I savored it fully, nibbling and sucking.

Stella moved down to her little black mound and nuzzled her face in it. I could tell she was tonguing her flower by the way Sabine was moaning. I continued to trace the tip of my tongue down the side of her ribs. I circled her belly button with my tongue, licking the inside slowly while fingering her nipples. I went down on her myself. It was the first time I had ever eaten a woman. Her pussy reminded me of a mango—the taste and texture was like an exotic fruit against my lips. I preferred sucking cock, cock, and more cock, in all its glory—but I kept at it. Then Stella brought Sabine to dripping wetness while she eased her fingers inside her cunt. Sabine arched back as the spasms of her orgasm took hold of her. I squeezed her nipples even harder while lunging my tongue in between her beautiful red lips. She gurgled in delight.

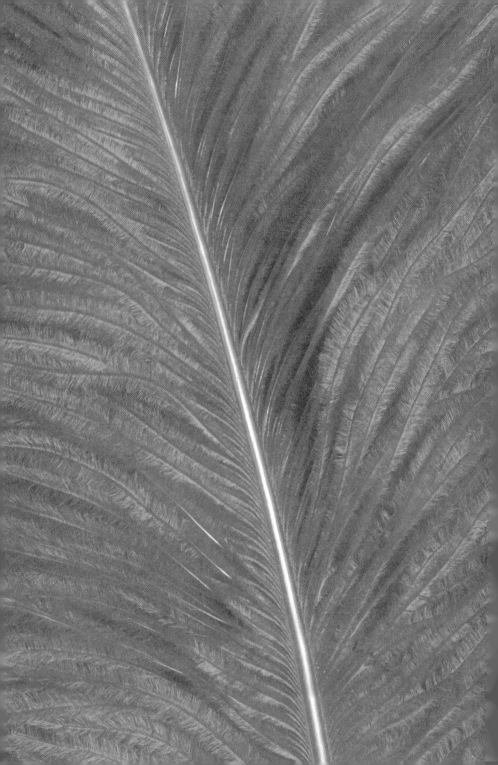

You May Kiss My Feet

Fetish fun . . .

Feet, glorious feet. However did they get the bad rap they have received in certain benighted quarters? Feet are among the most miraculous little devils on planet Earth—graceful, functional, mischievous, and infinitely sexy.

Sexy? And how. Even saying the word can cause a naughty little shiver to ripple down your spine. Try it slowly. *Fffff* . . . the teeth graze against the bottom lip in a manner that is both sweet and cruel. *Eeee* . . . Put 'em together with a pert little *t* at the close: *fffffeeeee . . . t!* Voila, you've got yourself a highly combustible end product, right down there at the end of your legs.

> The nerve endings for the genitals are right next to the foot in the body's brain maps.

Men with foot fetishes are very big in the dominatrix industry. They wanted me to use my feet in every way you could think of: slapping their dicks, smothering them with my day-old stockings, suffocating them till they nearly passed out, shoving my feet in their mouths till they gagged. They loved to stick their noses right under my steamy toes and take a deep, delirious whiff, give my arches a tongue bath and then paint my toenails scarlet, and have me dance on their noses. If you have never had your tootsies sucked, let me tell you it is heaven on earth. And the payoff? Let's just say it was not unusual for me to have to wash and sanitize my delicate peds after a session.

WHY FEET?

Because for some, feet represent the bottom, therefore the lowest, dirtiest, least desirable part of the human body. But that's precisely what gives them their kick. In the world of sex, up is often down, and nasty can be glorious. Who wants squeaky clean all the time? Don't we all want to exercise the parts of ourselves that like to be bad?

Consider this: Feet are regarded as bad mostly in America. We seem to have this antiseptic thing going on, and it robs our world of much of its zest. The rest of the planet still seems able to indulge their noses in what they're supposed to be indulging in. The Japanese were the first to climb this frontier. They understood the artistry of the foot that God created. In China, the exotic mildewed scent of a bound foot—like the finest mushroom—was one of its chief appeals. In Spain, flamenco dances have long showcased stamping feet, tightly encased in black clicking boots, to their best, most dangerously flashing effect. In Germany, well, have you ever spent time in German chat rooms? They're all about power, feet, and who can shove whose feet into whom. In France, natural God-given scents are relished with great anticipation like a fine perfume. In fact, in this connoisseur society where the nose ranks all wines and cheeses with the most sophisticated palate on earth, the highest compliment ever given to a big smelly blue cheese is to call it "the feet of God."

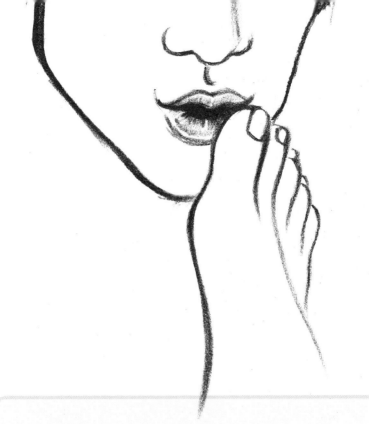

APPRECIATE YOUR PARTNER'S FETISH

If you're not initially attracted to a fetish, how do you become attuned to it?

I don't believe you can force a fetish on yourself. I advise that you be open to appreciating or enjoying various parts of the body. Crinkling your nose at someone's delicate feet can hurt his or her delicate ego. Do you really want to go there? In therapy, I worked with a husband who wanted his wife to dominate him. This was not an easy task, because ultimately all I could do was introduce the wife to the idea. In the end it was up to her to become open to it. It is all too easy to embarrass someone. The idea is to learn about different options and explore them to see if you like them or not. If they don't interest you, they don't interest you. But don't snub your nose at someone because you think their fetish is weird.

If you have a man with a genuine foot fetish, you win the big brass ring because there are so many ways to keep him interested. You can always tap into his fetish to revitalize his interest in you— just try waving your toes in front of his face and watch his eyes begin to blaze. Even American advertising is starting to wise up to the selling power of feet. (Notice how many ads no longer cut off the model at the bottoms of her ankles, so she can show off her tootsies? They're not dumb: They know that long after your breasts sag and your ass hangs, your feet will hold up as the reliable sex sparklers that they are.)

I adore having someone worship my arch, my heel, and the secret spaces between my toes. All those too-often-overlooked knobs and crevices crave an attention that is guaranteed to moisten my pussy.

HOW DO I FIND MY INNER FETISHES?

You don't. They find you. As a therapist, I have learned that people either have fetishes or they don't. They usually make themselves known to you by your early twenties. These predilections become like an itch that needs to be scratched. Scratch it in good health! Trying to ignore it (hello, repression?) can only cause a logjam somewhere else in your psyche.

One client lived to worship my feet. Tom was a thirty-nine-year-old political lobbyist, married with two children, who must have felt guilty about all his political dirty work because he loved nothing better than to roll around in submission at my feet. He said it "helped balance the scales of justice." For two years, I enjoyed

ILONA PARIS ON THE FOOT FETISH

*Feet are divine. Feet are pretty. Feet are elegant. American
women used to be embarrassed by their feet, but with
the pedicure revolution of the last several years we are
becoming more and more proud of them. Ultimately a woman
wants nothing more than for a man to acknowledge that he
loves her feet—preferably on his knees.*

*Fortunately, that's not hard to arrange, because it is
amazing how many men in our culture adore a woman's foot.
Oh, they profess to hate going into shoe stores, but with
the right kind of permission, they reveal that feet are one
of their most deeply hidden passions: the delicate arch,
the tips of our toes . . .*

*To a large extent, feet represent the last frontier in
female nudity. Think of how common T&A has become as
an icon of American salesmanship. You see breasts on
everything but cereal boxes. Yawn. But flaunt a little
toe cleavage in the park and watch those well-groomed
haircuts snap around. Let the double-takes begin.
Groveling is only a foot-length away.*

*For many pro Dommes, the Mistresses who are doing it for a
living, feet are the only part of their bodies they allow to
be touched. Their feet, powerful enough in their own right
(ever notice how strong those small muscles are?), thereby
obtain even more symbolic power. And that's not to mention*

coming up with creative ideas to torture and tease him. Tom usually
came late in the afternoon, often with the tiniest smirk on his face.
On one particular occasion, I opened the door and greeted him
with a walloping slap to the face. "Nice to see you, slave," I said
with a grin. I was wearing a bright green latex tank dress. I had

all those delectable little nerve endings down there, which reflexologists have claimed for centuries are the cure to most every ailment known to humankind.

For the woman who wants to spice up her own private love life, nothing could be finer. You get worship, a tongue bath, a reflexology massage, maybe even a pedicure rolled into one. Plus it's the most divinely calming sensation in the world—simultaneously soothing and subtly titillating. I dare you to find something else you can say that about. Go ahead, try it!

For a man who thinks he runs everything in life—who calls the board meeting and purchases the guest house—it can enhance his relation to his partner. Honoring the beauty of a woman creates a sensuous bond between a woman and man. Letting yourself go and not being afraid of where your passion takes you erotically helps to enhance creative loving. Like so much of this art, it is really about letting go of your fears.

But for the woman who knows how much she runs everything in life—who not only runs the boardroom and purchases the guest house, but also selects the summer camp and makes sure the fridge is stocked—the idea that she might be able to lie back while her lover takes control from the toes up can be more than seductive. It can be sanity-saving.

pulled my hair back and attached a long hairpiece that slid down over my shoulder. The dress just covered my vitals, and I let him get down on his knees to worship my feet. I wore six-inch crystal clear shoes so my red painted toenails could show themselves off in all their glory. The smirk was gone when he closed his eyes and inhaled my most private perfume, tinged with the earthiest of seasonings.

"I'm honored to be here, Mistress," he murmured.

"You should be, slave. Take off your clothes and get back down on your hands and knees. *Now!*" I whacked him again for good measure. He ripped his pants off and quickly got back down on the floor. I walked behind him and played with his balls with the tip of my shoe. My cat peered around the corner and purred. I scraped the heel of my stiletto along Tom's back. His head went back and he moaned in delight.

"Follow me, slave," I ordered.

> Dorothy knew what she was doing when she got those ruby slippers. But it was Glenda the Good Witch who had to teach her about them. Remember, you can be cruel to be kind.

I walked into my dungeon and sat in my tufted velvet throne, which rested upon a mirrored platform.

"Assume position, slut."

Tom kneeled with his hands clasped behind his back. I kicked open his knees. He knew that I liked the cock and balls to be available to me at all times. "Good boy," I said. "You may now kiss my feet."

I always liked to start a session this way. "You may use your hands," I added.

"Yes, Mistress."

He tentatively grasped the heel of my shoe as if it were the most precious object in the world. In his eyes, at that moment, my stilettoed foot was an object to be revered. Trembling with devotion, he leaned forward to kiss the tip. His hardness intensified as he planted kisses that felt like butterflies dancing on my toes. Towering over him, I watched him do this for a few minutes, cautiously at first, then with increasing hunger. He was literally swooning at my feet.

Submissives need to feel cleansed and released from the responsibilities of everyday life.

I said in my sternest voice, "Suck the heel of my shoe, slave. Give it a blow job." He gingerly placed the long six inches of my stiletto heel in his mouth. His tongue slathered along its deadly length until it shone. A man of this stature needed an outlet to release him from all the responsibilities in his life, and he obviously relished giving himself over to me. I sat back in my chair admiring the scenery.

"You may take off my shoe." (For your information, I would never walk around barefoot in front of a client. My stilettos were similar to Samson's hair in the Bible. They were what gave me my power. I never traveled far from them!)

He did so, relishing the softness of my skin, the slight clamminess of my soles. He sensed the change my aroma brought to the air, the charge it brought to our proceedings. I let him have his way with my feet, understanding that it was like nourishment to him. Due to protocol, I would only let him go so far, but I imagined him savoring their loveliness, their allure and pull. In my mind he devoured my long toes, licking between, under, and around each one, sucking my soles and swallowing my heels. How many times had this been done to me in real life, with real-life lovers, as they inhaled deeply, nibbling softly into the ball of my foot, the chaste flesh just beneath the dollops of my digits, the juiciest part of my sole that was like paradise to them?

"Show me who's boss, Mistress," he whimpered. "Punish me for all the terrible things I do."

All right, I don't mind if I do. Very gingerly I planted my slender

THE CARE AND FEEDING OF A FOOT FETISH

Giving someone a foot bath and massage is all about service. Think of yourself as being back in the Roman ages. You—or ideally, your partner—are a servant determined to give the best service to your Mistress. You are there to please. Here is what I recommend:

Start off with the right implements. To begin, invest in a special foot bathtub—a simple plastic one from your local CVS or Kmart will do (though the fancier the better, obviously, because we're talking about making the event special. Those vibrating tubs can be wonderful.) Next, pour warm water into the tub. Add a fragrant bubble bath such as lavender or rose petal. Honey or almond are wonderful scents for aromatherapy. You can use something from Chanel or go to your health food store and use any of the products from Kiss My Face. A scented candle is nice, too.

Put the Mistress' or Master's peds in the tub. Sprinkle rose petals all over the water. Slowly soap her feet with a French milled soap or Trader Joe's Rose Petal soap. Take a pumice stone or pumice-like instrument and rub underneath the foot and on the edges of the foot, particularly the

foot, my elegant appendage, square on his face.

How his skin stretched back under my arch! How he struggled to breathe under my fragrant toes! This was the same face that had smirked at me when it came through the door, and now it was anti-smirking! It was regretting any insolence it had ever shown me, or had shown any woman, for that matter.

After I'd released Tom from my toes, I put a white ruffled apron on him and told him to crawl into my kitchen while I buffed my nails. (My square manicure was getting unruly.) Tom always brought the

heel area. This is a sensitive area, so gauge what feels good. Treat the heel like it's the most beautiful object in the world. Make sure you run a finger slowly between each toe. This feels soooooo good. Then take succulent grapes and drop them in the bottom of the tub. Have your sweetie smush her toes in the grapes. It provides a delightful feeling underneath the feet that is quite unexpected. Lift her feet out and rub them in a warmed towel.

Of course, even if you've done all this with the best accoutrements in the world, if you don't have a spectacular technique in handling her feet, the effect will be ruined. So pay special attention now. Take a richly thick lotion or oil and massage her toes with it. Rub the heels, then go up and down the arch. Circle around the pads of the foot. Then do each toe with as much love and attention as you can. Don't rush it! Lavish tenderness on each toe as if your life depended on it. This is an act of generosity on your part. Do it with love. Finally, wrap the feet in the heated towel and hold them with your hands so the heat from your body comes through.

most expensive chocolate as a gift to me, and this session had been no exception. I asked him to melt it—he'd be licking it off my toes soon enough. "Don't make a mess!" I reminded him.

The Godiva "G" collection, made from premium cocoa beans in such flavors as Tasmanian Honey and Mexican Hot Chocolate, needed to be just syrupy enough to pour. Pour I did—once he had brought it to me, and I had him lying down at the base of my throne, with his wrists attached by cuffs and his feet locked to a spreader bar—right over my arch. His mouth was planted below, so his tongue caught each molten drop as it dripped between my toes. *Ahh*, I loved the sensation of having a footboy lick expensive chocolate ($120 per pound) from my feet. Nothing but the best, but then, he was paying good money for this experience ($250 per hour).

PLAYTIME: **PLAY TREASURE HUNT WITH YOUR TOES**

Make him lie down on the floor beneath you and use your toes to locate the invisible treasure on his face. Grasp it with your toes. Dig in a bit with your nails. Is it his nose? His eyebrows? His chin? His lips? His ears? You'll never find the invisible treasure because it doesn't exist, but you'll both have fun hunting.

Once my feet were clean again, and I had unfastened Tom from his restraints, our session was almost done. "Would you like a release, slave?" I asked.

He silently begged me with his eyes until I handed him a little towel and informed him he could jerk himself off—but only by watching my feet. I stepped over to my leopard-skinned chair, ever

Embarrassed?
People sometimes worry because they can't
understand where these fetishes come from and
are afraid to share them with their loved ones.
Lighten up!
Be open to your lover's desires or try to find
something you are both comfortable with.

so leisurely put on a favorite pair of shoes (Christian Laboutins that
were so hot I never knew whether to wear them or to fuck them),
and with half-closed eyes sat back to watch the show.

As Tom stroked his cock, I very slowly crossed and uncrossed
my legs. He stared at the lines of toe cleavage, remembering that
these divine toes were recently in control of his existence. I let the
shoe dangle off my foot, causing him to moan. "Look nowhere else,"
I commanded, "and remember that you must ask for permission
before you come." His movements became quicker and the skin on
his face began to tighten. His cock turned a deep purple and looked
as if it was about to explode.

"May I come, Mistress?"

"Not quite yet," I purred.

He stared at my feet, grunting in frustration and desire.

"Please, Mistress, please."

"No."

"Please, Mistress, please!"

"Oh, all right."

Right on cue, he released himself and let out sigh after sigh. I
stood to my full height before him as his trembling diminished and

ILONA PARIS ON FETISHES

A crucial distinction: there are fetishes for material objects such as latex or leather, and there are fetishes of the body. In this chapter we focus on the latter—body parts that bring a glint to your eye, make your nostrils flare, and elicit moisture between your legs or the tip of your penis.

Fetishes are a delight. Unfortunately, our culture has made people embarrassed about that which they ought to delight in. Our society seems to feel it will lose control if we go for what it claims is not normal. I feel we need to honor the body and pursue that which ignites passion within ourselves and where we find beauty. Americans are so afraid to let go. But if we use our senses, they are like wonderful gifts bestowed upon our bodies that are limitless in the doors they can open.

When are fetishes unhealthy? They are unhealthy when they take over our lives, when they hurt us mentally or physically, or do the same to someone else. A fetish has the potential to become an addiction, and that is where it becomes tricky. Enjoy your fetish, appreciate and nourish it, but don't get swallowed up by it. It is a part of your life—but not all of it. See the difference?

Another point worth making: Fetishes keep you interested. I mean, tits and ass are fine as far as they go, but who wants a steady diet of T&A? Thus the expression "vanilla"—how boring. It's like having oatmeal day after day. Feet, armpits, hair, the back of the neck, pubic hair—all these fetishes add spice to a diet that could otherwise be bland. That's why I call fetishes the salt and pepper of the sex world. We have all these wonderful parts of the body—why not enjoy them?

So imagine settling back into the ottoman and having your shoes removed by caring hands. Having manly knuckles pressed lovingly into your arch, then your toes firmly squeezed, one after the other. Slowly he lowers his head to your feet. Adoringly he opens his mouth to take your baby toe between his lips. You close your eyes and swoon with the sensations about to be bestowed upon you . . .

finally subsided entirely. Once again I noted how similar a good domination session was to a good therapy session: both left the client feeling deeply at peace with himself. Tom was at rest, in his body and his mind. He smiled.

I smiled back. "You may kiss my foot to show your appreciation," I gently ordered.

He was on his knees, hands clasped behind his back, and bent over to kiss the top of my shoe and bare toes. I placed my hand on the top of his head and stated, "That is the end of your session. You may get dressed."

"Suffice it to say that submission in a D/S context is one of the rare times when the revelation of one's deepest and most forbidden sexual desires is not merely tolerated but is lovingly encouraged and rewarded."

—*Brame and Brame*

I walked out of the dungeon into my living room to let him get changed. It was my turn to relax. I sat down in my purple shell-shaped chair, stifled a yawn, and waited for his departure.

Hard work being a goddess, but someone had to do it.

BLOW MY HEEL

If the idea of having someone suck on your stiletto doesn't do much for you, there is a world of opportunity when it comes to feet. Here are some suggestions:

- Invite your partner to go shoe shopping. Wear a sexy dress and make sure your toes are perfectly pedicured. Slowly try on shoes, showing your toe cleavage. If this sounds too time-consuming, pretend to shop in your very own closet. Oh, and I would highly suggest wearing a see-through dress.

- Tie your partner up and paint his or her toes—he'll think of you as he sits behind his desk with ruby red toenails inside his shoes.

- Have your partner tie you down and make love to your toes with his or her mouth.

- Ask your partner for a foot massage, preferably in the nude, while you're watching television—you may just have to shut off the set before American Idol ends.

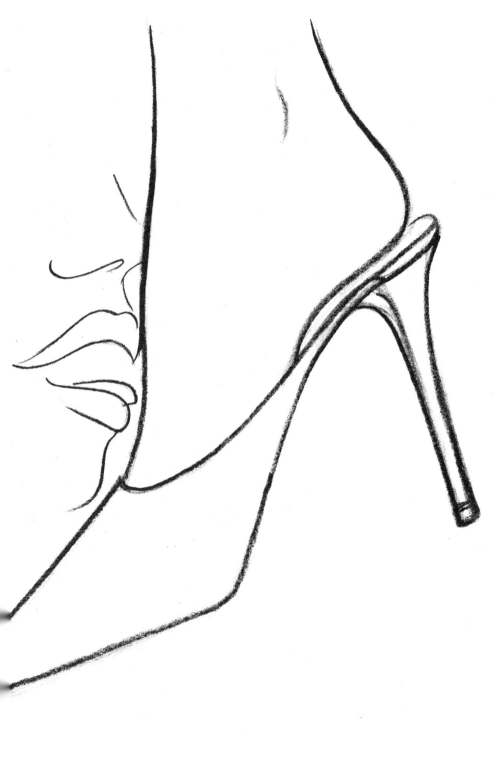

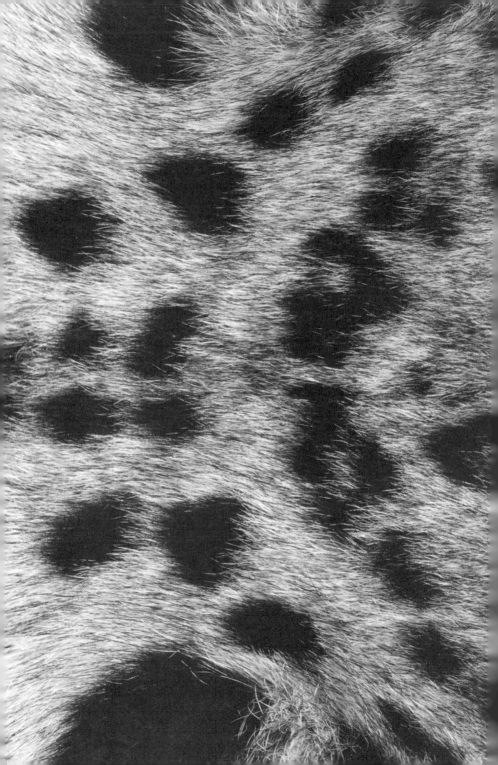

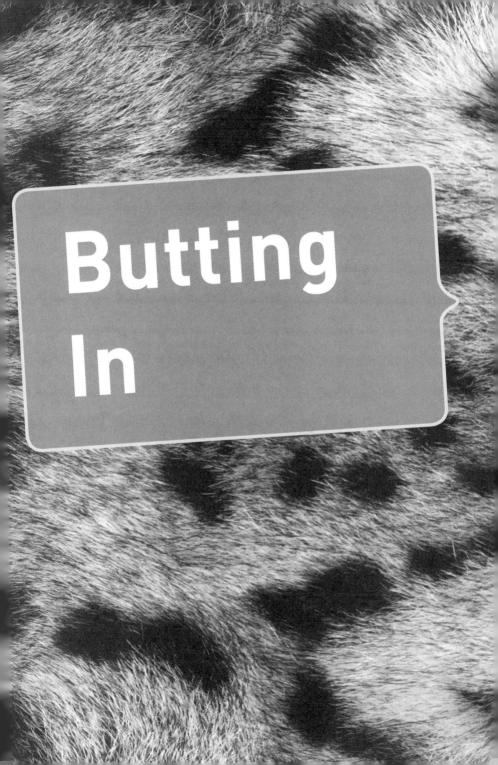

Butting In

The black hole in your own backyard.

Okay, time for me to blush.

A dark confession.

Loath as I am to admit it—and I won't blame you if you stop your ears—for all my experimentation, there was one hole I was a little late in filling. Well, not that late—it just wasn't the first thing on my mind. Anal sex wasn't talked about in those days. Besides, I was so busy having every other kind of sex that I never got around to it. But once I discovered it, I never looked back, so to speak. It became part and parcel of my overall sexual repertoire. Today, with the right person, anal sex is one of many ways I fulfill myself. Let me tell you how I discovered the hole in my own backyard.

Ever read Toni Bentley's book, *The Surrender*? She caused a scandal du jour by maintaining that anal sex is better than vaginal. Well, you'd better find out for yourself, hadn't you?

For a while I specialized in going out by myself. The reason was simple: I could get into more trouble that way. One night I found my way to a tiny basement jazz club—a dark little joint right in the middle of the sleepy

34 percent of men and 30 percent of women said they had tried anal sex.
—Survey of 12,000 people by National Survey of Family Growth

little Boston suburb of Athol, Massachusetts. (I kid you not—the name drew me like a moth to a flame.) I was wearing a wonderful, expensive black suit, black hose, and a white silk blouse. My hair was in a French twist. I looked, shall we say, enticing. In about forty seconds a man circled around me like a panther, smooth and sleek. My God, this man was the ultimate in eye candy. He was tall, at least six-foot-two, and was wearing a smooth black suit. He had the most beautifully heart-shaped face with high, high cheekbones. His eyes were the shape of large almonds, brown and soft. His lips were beautiful and full. The first words that came out of those luscious lips were, "You must be married."

"No, why?" I said.

"Anyone as beautiful as you must be married."

It worked. Winston—let's call him Winston—asked me to dance, and when we got to the dance floor, I relaxed in a way I rarely had before. Dancing always relaxed me anyway, but this time I felt a special looseness. The club was throbbing with beautiful bodies dancing to incredible funky music, and my man could move. He had a way of putting his hand by his dick when he was dancing. It looked like he was holding himself. His sexual energy was sucking me in like a pool of quicksand while I watched. I couldn't get away even if I'd wanted to.

DIFFERENT SURRENDERS

Sexual preferences are not set in stone. They're fluid, changing over time. Some people get off reading Tolstoy when they're in college. Later in life it might be Anne Rice's vampire scenes that get them hot. Flow with it.

"I knew only as we pounded suddenly into the middle of the road, that I was drenched in shame, each marching step intensifying it, and yet I felt as I always did at the core of punishment; the coming of a tranquility, a quiet place in the very center of frenzy, in which I could surrender all the parts of my being."
— A. N. Roquelaure, Beauty's Punishment

Winston knew how to play with a woman. He taunted, he teased, he titillated. He had a deep laugh that was just infectious. He also had an allure—I don't know how to put it—the promise of a darker kind of eroticism than I was accustomed to. Something mysterious and a little scary. It made me want to catch him and hang on for dear life. But we were still on the dance floor. How was I going to get him into my lair?

Oh yeah, Shirley. Thank God for my yellow bug machine.
We put-putted over to my apartment. Needless to say he was a pleasure to kiss. Those plump lips of his gave me something to bite into. I think we kissed on my bed for hours. It was like eating fine caviar, tiny bit by tiny bit. Finally he found my neck and lavished it with his warm, soft tongue. I quivered at the tantalizing sensation. He reached my clavicle and gently ran his tongue across it. It felt like I was being tickled with some sort of antique quill, soft and sharp at the same time. When he finally reached

my breast, I was moaning unintelligibly. He passed over it with feather-like strokes. Meanwhile he was rubbing the tip of my other nipple between his fingers. He then nibbled its twin with his teeth, flicking the tip of his tongue in between bites.

"Good shame can lead to self-discovery and growth and can nurture and protect it while bad shame humiliates and makes you feel bad about the way you look or feel."

— Dr. Joyce Brothers

Getting lost in this man's body was a delight. I started to peel away his clothes and it was like peeling away the skin of an exotic fruit. His skin was a lightly dusted cocoa. His chest was full and ripe, while his legs were ready to be eaten. His butt was like two perfect grapefruits. Enough with the fruit, I needed to move on to the pastry. His cock was fabulous. I was a happy girl as I put my mouth on it and savored its sweetness. It was too beautiful to do anything else. The tight black curly pubic hair surrounding it made it all the more enticing. I wanted it and I wanted all of it.

He was as enchanted by my body as I was by his. My skin, especially. He kept repeating how soft my skin was. He seemed to be mesmerized by the silkiness of my flesh and exclaimed that he couldn't get enough. This is music to a woman's ears; at least it was to mine.

He gradually worked his way down to my stomach, then to my pussy. This man had a tongue from heaven. He knew how to flick it perfectly over my clit, bringing me to new heights of intensity. He lifted my knees and pushed them up and over so that my asshole was totally exposed to him.

Bells started going off. Sort of a combination of alarm bells, wedding bells, and every other kind. I was feeling every sort of emotion at once. Was I afraid? Ashamed? Of my own anus? My curiosity was at warp speed. Let's just say I wanted to get to the bottom of things. On the one hand, I loved the feeling of just totally giving myself up to receive pleasure. Of being exposed like that, split open like a piece of ripe melon, open to whatever might come.

On the other hand, I was petrified of that thing going up my ass and hurting me. I won't lie. The idea of it filling my most untested hole made me pant a little. I mean, I'd always assumed that in my world every orifice was game, but now that I was up against it . . .

Winston was very patient with me, and I found myself surrendering. I lay back and breathed deeply into what I was about to receive. He "went around the world," licking the rim of my anus so that my hole naturally expanded for him to shove his tongue all the way in. He went back to titillating my clitoris so that spasms of electricity started to emanate from my little pearl. Currents of warmth pulsed through my labia until the overwhelming rush of an orgasm followed. His face glistened in the candlelight. What, you think I didn't have candles all around my bed, ready for any sex urgency?

AROUND THE WORLD

A woman loves to have her anus licked. (Well, I do.) Remember that a woman likes to be teased almost anywhere. Foreplay can never be prolonged enough. Let your partner gently explore your nether regions. Relax into the new sensations you are about to experience. Literally try to be open to it.

Is heterosexual anal sex more popular with Generation X? Statistics from *Playboy* and the Kinsey Institute Surveys indicate that a generational change has occurred whereby people born in the last two decades are more comfortable having, or at least admitting to having, anal sex than earlier generations.

We rested a moment, and then he produced a tube of Vaseline. I guess he carried around a supply for his own sex urgencies. He had me stand in front of him and bend over. Slowly he spread my ass cheeks. It was the most submissive and vulnerable position I had ever found myself in. I could feel the coolness of the evening air against my tender opening. Exposing your asshole to someone is the ultimate in vulnerability. You are out there 100 percent. This was an extremely electric moment. I was scared shitless, but I was feeling my body buzzing in anticipation at the same time.

After he rubbed the Vaseline very slowly around my anus, he stood up behind me. He had the most beautifully smooth abdomen and powerful legs I had ever seen. He started to put the tip of his penis in my ass. I was tight as a clam. It hurt, and I started to whine. To his eternal credit, he was kind, gentle, and patient. He showed me that I had to work through it. While my mini leopard, Sushi, went bonkers on the other side of the room (jealous, honey?), Winston pushed a little bit and waited for me to push back against him, tentatively at first and then, slowly, with growing confidence. He kept pushing and pushing and then pulling back a little. The nerve endings in this part of my body started going crazy; it was like they were waking up after a long sleep.

The most amazing sensations coursed through me. I could feel his cock swathed in heat right through my rectum. After a

ILONA PARIS ON ANAL SEX

Though I was a bit freaked out the first time it happened, anal sex is now one of my personal masturbation fantasies. It feels wonderful and it affords the absolute end-all in terms of intimacy with another human being. Allowing yourself to let go from this central spot can be a total release, leaving you with a sense of having accomplished something profound and developing a deeper sense of intimacy. It can be a wonderful moment for you as an individual and as a couple.

But anal sex is a touchy subject for a lot of people—not only physically but psychologically. The Catholic Church during the Middle Ages deemed that anal sex was a sin and in some strange way that frame of mind continues today. It's bad enough for people to enjoy sex—but to openly proclaim their pleasure in receiving anal intercourse? Hellfire.

Straight men tend to shudder at the notion of receiving anal sex. Gay men are into it, of course, but mention it to a straight man who is not open to his sexuality, and he either turns his head the other way or makes a silly joke about the fudge factor.

The truth is that all people have the capacity to enjoy anal sex. Really. Men, both gay and straight, can take as much pleasure in it as women. When I was a dominatrix the most

while it was like my nerves were stretching and gripping and clamoring for more. I was like an animal in heat—never more vulnerable, never more turned on. My ego was forgotten, and I was all physical being, demanding my pleasure be slaked. The fear factor was gone; there was just the "want factor" as in "I want it up there!" And there it was!

common question clients asked in their initial interview was if I performed anal sex with a strap-on. That was my big revelation about my straight male clients—they liked to be fucked up the ass—and with a good six inches, if you please.

Women tend to get all bashful and virginal when the subject arises. It's as if we can't 'fess up to desiring or craving this particular pleasure, like let's all ignore the giant pink dildo in the middle of the living room. Even for me, your all-experienced sexpert, it was hard to imagine in the beginning that sex in this manner could feel so wonderfully hot. Now I expect my lover to be experienced in this area.

Here's what I suggest: that we all settle down and get used to the fact that anal sex is here to stay. Not only is there nothing wrong with it; we should celebrate the fact that we have this glorious hole to be enjoyed and titillated. Some of the most sensitive nerve endings are in the anus. You can't tell me God created it just so it feels good when we go to the bathroom. So take a deep breath and proclaim with me: "Hail, hail to the asshole for one and for all!"

As the Marquis de Sade once said, "Have done with virtues! Among the sacrifices that can be made to those counterfeit divinities, is there one worth an instant of the pleasures one tastes in outraging them?"

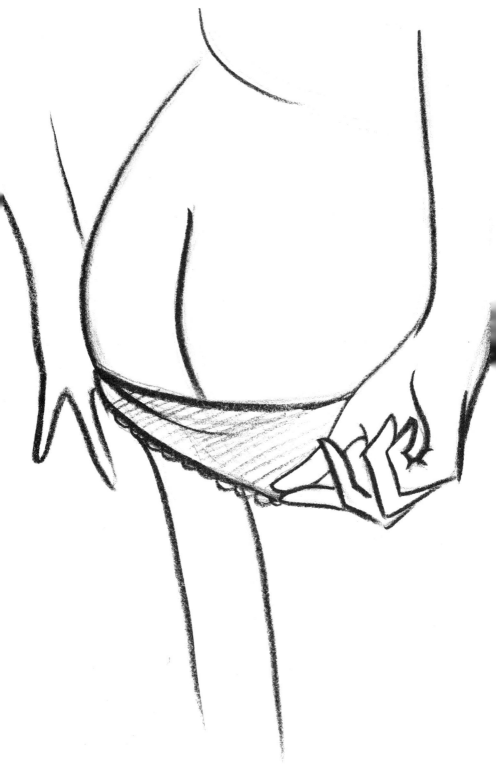

THE CARE AND FEEDING OF THE GLORIOUS ANUS

Allowing someone to enter my most private of spaces is the ultimate in closeness. Despite my wild and crazy life, it is not something I just give to anyone, and they have to know what they are doing. Someone who just rams his cock up my ass can walk right out the door as far as I am concerned.

Here's what he or she has to know: a lot of foreplay is necessary. You want the person to excite you so that you are dripping and sweating from every place your body can possibly be dripping and sweating. Every inch of you needs to be worked over so you are totally loose and relaxed. An expert lover will gradually slide his or her fingers up your ass in such a way that you welcome it and receive it. Once your partner has you totally relaxed and wanting more, the rectum should be ready to open further. With lots of lube he should slowly work his way into your canal.

One precaution: the anus must be honored and cared for. Not only must you approach it tenderly and with compassion, but you also need to be aware of the hygiene factor. The anus is where we relieve ourselves of our excrement. Therefore it provides an environment where a lot of germs can thrive. Whether it's a penis, a dildo, fingers, or mouth, never go from the anus into the vagina without first washing well. Keep sanitizer lotion by the bed for your hands, but be careful not to let the lotion come into contact with your delicate genital areas (it stings!). After the deed is done and you're happily purring with contentment, don't forget to wash up with soap and water. Do the same with any toys you are using.

Remember, also, that the tissue in your anus is especially delicate. You have to take measures to avoid ripping or scratching it. That's one of the reasons why you always want to use a condom and always, always use lubricant. The other reason is that a condom helps prevent the exchange of blood and bodily fluids—particularly if you are with someone you don't know well. Before you engage in anal sex, take an STD or AIDS test if you haven't done so already. Not a bad policy for any sexual activity, for that matter.

A Strap-On Birthday Party

I was once invited to a birthday party that a well-known dominatrix
threw for her favorite slave. The slave's fantasy was to have all the
women at the party fuck her with a strap-on dildo. I had never
done this before and was a bit concerned. I didn't want to hurt her.
Silly me!

> At parties or by myself, sometimes it hits me:
> Why use drugs like Ecstasy or coke when we have
> such deeper resources within ourselves?

I arrived at the party with my companion, a Dom who was well
known for his torturous antics with his submissives. The house
was a little gray and white ranch on Cape Cod. We walked in to see
an interesting array of people: some were clothed in bizarre fetish
attire, while one sissy maid wore a red Shirley Temple wig with a
full set of petticoats. Slaves ran around wearing nothing but black
leather thongs. I liked this look the best.

The birthday slave was a young elfin woman in her thirties,
who was very nondescript. Her arms and legs were skinny, her hair
was a bland blond, and her eyes were a washed-out blue. Nothing
about her announced that she was an outrageous pig who wanted
everyone in the room to fuck her up the ass. While waiting for the
main event I sat on the rug and made out with a transvestite. Well,
it was something to do, and she did have soft lips.

At last, a leather-covered sawhorse was brought out for the
birthday girl. Various women had brought their own strap-ons in
all sorts of decorative colors and sizes. One dildo was a swirl of
green and black, while another was a Day-Glo hot pink number.

The Mistress of the house lent me one of hers, a purple job with knobs that would fit up the anal canal nicely. A tall, strong male slave with a spectacular set of legs—all three—offered to guide me through the process. He helped me fit the straps around my waist and legs. Making sure the strap-on is secure, I learned, is of utmost importance. You don't want it slipping all over the place. We then put a condom on it for extra protection. This was new to me because I'd always thought you could just wash the thing off afterward. He poured a pool of personal lubricant in my hand, and after I lathered up, I was good to go.

I had the honor of going first. The slave's creamy white derriere waited in anxious anticipation. Her rosebud of an anus was exposed. I swear it kind of winked at me, waiting for me to deflower it. I stood behind her in my five-inch black laced platform boots. Thank God, I had a sturdy foundation. Doing this in stilettos would have made me more than a little wobbly.

RAISING THE ILONA FACTOR

Remember that many men love to have a strap-on dildo used on them. Lesbians have known the delights of strap-ons for years. Why not men? As a dominatrix, I found men regularly asked for this. Give him a nice, sturdy six inches, ladies, and watch him roar.

The slave lay on the sawhorse with her derriere extended, welcoming me to dip the tip of the dildo in her well-lubricated anus. This was a woman who was used to anal sex so she wasn't overly tight. Cautiously I slipped it into the opening and began to feel my way in. Being the slut she was, she seemed to almost

"We throw around the term 'sexual
desire' as though we're all sure
we're talking about the same thing.
But it's clear from the research that
people have very different operational
definitions about what desire is."

—Lisa M. Diamond, psychologist at the University of Utah

sigh with relief. Some onlookers were *oohing* and *ahhing*, but I was
so into what I was doing that everything and everyone became a
colorful blur around me. It was as if I had entered my own private
Idaho. I was very sensitive to gradually working this woman's cavity
so it stayed relaxed. A drop of sweat ran between my breasts.
After a minute or two I was able to sense a groove with my hips. I
developed an instinct about how far I could push into her. When
I got it, I started to fuck her royally. All of a sudden I felt like Wonder
Woman, riding a magnificent white horse and watching the ripples
of her beautiful back beneath me. I understood why women like
horseback riding so much. Who knew that one could experience
so much power from such a little space!

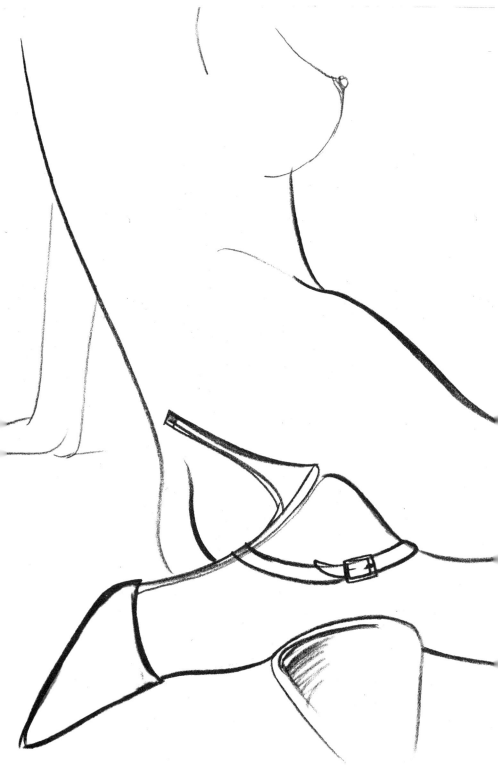

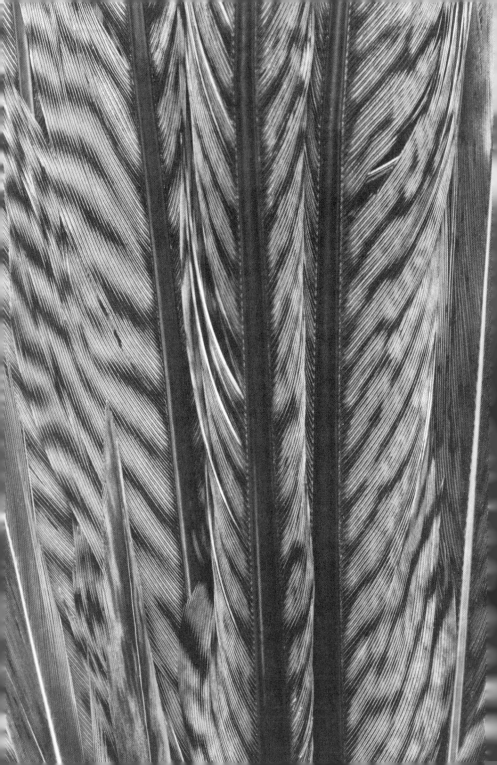

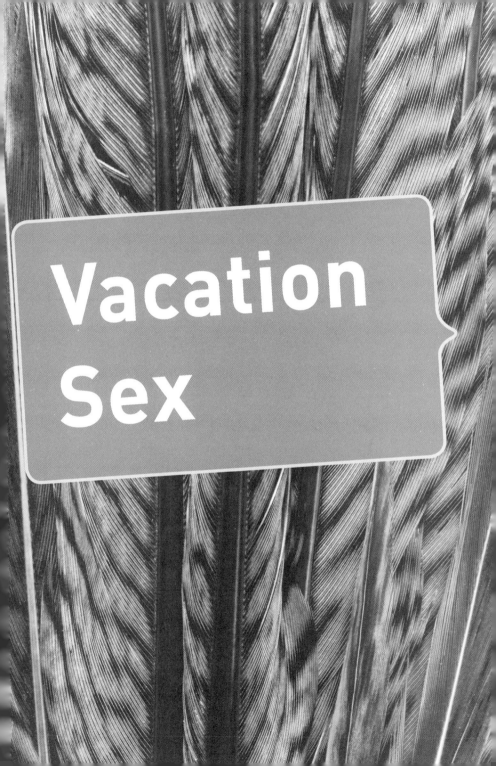

Sometimes it's good to step back and observe the scene around you. Who knows what tricks you might pick up?

Not quite ready to build your own dungeon? Unable to delve into naughty sex while your little ones are asleep in the next room? I suggest a change of scenery. (And not just of your nether regions!) You need a vacation, my darling. A vacation in which all bets are off. Anything goes. The sky's the limit. You know why? It's time for that best of all inventions: vacation sex!

Oh yes, vacations are the time I like to experiment with something altogether new. As a respite from the daily grind, they help me perfect my sense of self and come up with a new and improved, even more devious Ilona. Not only does this help recharge my batteries and give me valuable perspective on myself and the glorious world of sex, sometimes it even gives me fresh new naughtiness to take home. The trick is to be prepared but at the same time not to expect anything at all. That's when something exciting will usually happen. Don't try to force anything, but lie back, relax, and be open to anything that awaits you.

Anything, anything at all.

Hedonism Resort

Time for the show! It was another night in Jamaica at a festival called "Kink in the Caribbean." Suspense was high because the performer, Dita Von Teese, the infamous fetish model, was rarely seen. She stayed inside her suite during daylight hours so the sun did not touch her lily white skin. Only occasionally did we get a glimpse of her slipping out for a smoke wearing a vintage black and white polka-dot dress and a black straw hat right out of Sandra Dee's closet from the fifties. I had seen her on the cover of so many S&M magazines I could have creamed in my pants. Here she was now doing her world-famous fetish striptease, and that was just the evening's warm-up!

Pretend that your partner is a stranger
you just picked up at a bar—and that your husband
is watching you. This will push all kinds
of buttons on both of you: voyeurism, jealousy,
and some that don't even have names!

I first heard about "Kink" from a flyer I found among the vendors at the Fetish Flea Market in Boston, promising a fun-filled no-holds-barred week in the sun to take place at a pink and yellow resort called Hedonism III on the beach in Jamaica. Photos on their Website showed titillating scenes: a human table with sushi and glitter all over a woman's naked body; a Mistress in a captain's cap sassily submerging her black-latexed slave in a swimming pool. The festival featured daily workshops on bondage, singletail whips, medical play, and the like. They also had kinky Olympics with such feats as tying up your slave with the best hog tie, pony races, and turning your slave into an ice-cream sundae. A dungeon suite was open twenty-four hours a day for people to play in. How long do you think it took me to sign up?

CAN'T AFFORD THE AIRFARE?

Hedonism III is truly an Ilona-ized vacation treat. But if there don't happen to be sushi-laden human tables at your getaway resort, customize! Just getting out of your element into the privacy of a hotel can go a long way toward helping you get zany.

Here's how to create your own Caribbean getaway at the local no-tell motel: Reserve a king-sized bed. Light the candles around the room and have a platter of exotic fruit such as mangoes, bananas, and pineapple. Pour some sangria. Start by sipping from each other's glasses. Proceed to feeding each other chunks of pineapple with your fingers. Tease him by deep-throating your banana while eating it. You may dip his cock in your beverage and suckle it for a new exotic cocktail. Then sit on the edge of the bed and place your favorite fruit in your pussy so that it sticks out just enough for your lover to "swim" between your legs and have his delight. I have always adored having a man eat food from my pussy because then when he is done he can just keep on going with the real thing.

Lucky for me, I didn't have to pretend. Strangers were everywhere. At the grass-thatched dining room, I ran into three cosmopolitan chaps. Hans from Amsterdam was wearing black leather pants with a beautiful draping silk shirt. Ian from London had on a bizarre black leather vest akin to what an avenger of Spartacus might have worn, with matching cape, black knee-high boots with silver metal wings, and a singletail whip curled around his left shoulder. It was hard to miss his belt buckle, a writhing snake staring me in the face. Tall, Swedish-born Klaus, with long golden-brown hair that came to his shoulders, wore nothing but leather panties with a little flogger and handcuffs attached to his belt.

We all grabbed plates and sat down to a delightful dinner of squid pancakes and Caribbean lobster. After dinner we relaxed with coffee and drinks as the lights were turned down. Throbbing music started to pulsate as Fritz the ringmaster—bald, stocky, with a top hat—blew fire several feet into the air from his mouth. The moment had arrived for Dita Von Teese to perform. Stagehands carried out a sexy purple velvet divan surrounded by gauzy material. This was followed by some very slow, sexy music. Into the spotlight stepped Miss Von Teese. A chuff of amazement escaped from everyone sitting there.

Drop-dead gorgeous, she resembled a cross between Natalie Wood and Gypsy Rose Lee. Her jet-black hair was sculpted into a Veronica Lake pageboy along the sides of her face, and her lips were painted in a perfect red pout. She wore a glorious pink silk and satin corset tied with pink ribbons in the back. A pink tulle skirt puffed out around her hips, accentuating her teeny corseted waist. She even wore a matching bonnet tied with pink ribbons underneath her chin. The pièce de résistance were the pink toe shoes covered in fake diamonds. She stepped to and fro and twirled on her toes, posing. Slowly she removed her long satin gloves and slithered out of her skirt. As we hooted and gasped, she proceeded to undo the pink

> "Some people have to be tied up to be free."
>
> —Charles Moser, Ph.D., M.D., of the Institute for Advanced Study of Human Sexuality in San Francisco

ribbons on her back and remove her corset. Eventually Dita was wearing only a little diamond-studded G-string, half obscured by two giant pink ostrich feather fans delicately held in front and back. Lying back on her purple divan, she reminded me of a piece of puff pastry on an elegant piece of Limoges. After the show, an island bonfire party had been planned for us on the beach. Kicking off my six-inch stilettos, I left my companions and strolled the few steps to the sand. A stage had been set up for fire-blowers, and various torture apparatus had been scattered here and there under the palm trees.

Mistress Torturella was there with her slave, Tom. Their agreement was that, in return for the honor of paying for her trip, he would be tortured throughout the week by his Mistress. Torturella was a Rubenesque blond with catlike green eyes, a sweet woman with a quirky sense of humor. She made Tom get down on his hands and knees and suck the purple dildo she had strapped to her black leather corset. He was wearing nothing but a black leather thong. I like a man in a thong. I think they should all wear them in their spare time. She asked if I would like to play with her slave. How could I refuse?

ONE FOR ME, ONE FOR YOU

Reciprocity is the ticket. Let him know that what's good for him is also good for you. I always love it when a man goes to the trouble of trimming his pubic hair and putting powder or cologne on his private area. Drives me crazy. In return, it's only natural for me to think of what can I do to drive him crazy.

CLOSER TO HOME

You don't have to go far to discover a new side to your libido. Sometimes just getting out of the house will do it. How about hitting your local Home Depot with no underwear? Find a nice power tool. Then ask a big man how to use it.

I grabbed his hair and dragged him across the sand to a cross that was set up on the beach. I slapped black leather handcuffs to his wrists and clipped them onto the cross's hooks.

"Spread your legs, slut," I ordered.

Spying a coconut on the beach, I carefully placed it between his legs and told him to hold it there or else he would be severely punished. We were starting to draw a crowd. Exhibitionism for both the slave and the Mistress can be a fun thing when doing a scene in public. I traced my blood-red nails slowly from the tops of his shoulders all the way down to the backs of his legs, leaving subtle scratch trails all over his back. I walked around to look in his eyes. I took a big sip of water from my cup and spit it into his face, then for punctuation, took a handful of the cool beach sand and let it cascade over his back and shoulders. Everyone watching gave me a round of applause.

As I was soaking up the sights, something caught my attention out of the corner of my eye. On the beach not twenty yards away, a Mistress named Lady Eville and her 300-pound sidekick, Brunhilda, had managed to plastic wrap a submissive male to a palm tree. They had used so much wrap that he looked like a giant-sized caterpillar larva, stuck and helpless in the moonlight. A straw had been inserted into his mouth so he could breathe. Left exposed were his nipples, as well as his cock and balls, so that clamps could be attached to these sensitive areas. He could do nothing but whimper—truly an example of torture at its most elegant.

I migrated to a nearby pool and made the acquaintance of a Scotsman named Zak and his wife, who were in their early fifties and very pleasant. However, "pleasant" wasn't what interested me. It was Zak's serious rubber fetish—he was turned on by the feel of the material against his skin—which he had apparently been hiding from his wife until a year before. The fact that she was here at the event was a big deal for them both. Zak had a rubber body bag, in which he could float and experience

> "The satisfaction gained from S&M is something far more than sex. It can be a total emotional release."
>
> —Roy Baumeister, Ph.D., social psychologist at Case Western Reserve University

the sensation of being encased in rubber while submersed in the water. Now this was something one couldn't do in one's little old dungeon at home. We inflated the bag with a vacuum pump so he would float, zipped him into it, and rolled him into the water with a plop. I grabbed some purple rope, and we pulled him around the entire pool, pouncing on him, pushing him under the water, and making him pop up like a whale. He was loving the very new distorted physical sensations he was experiencing. This was all new to his wife, and she was a bit blown away, but she tentatively tried to help. Little by little she got into the game, until she, too, was slapping the bag and having a grand old time. Plainly, this vacation was as therapeutic for her as any session I could have provided in my office.

Thus warmed up, it was time to check out the dungeon. As if sensing an invisible signal, everyone else apparently had the same idea, and from all corners of the resort bodies slunk forth, newly leathered up.

LEATHER UP

Animal rights activists have a noble cause, but they're never going to convert kinksters away from the use of leather. Nothing beats leather for its dark, soft, and supple qualities. Nor can any synthetic substitute possibly smell so animalistic. When someone is dressed in black leather you feel this person is mysterious, dangerous, and ready for the dark side—evil, rebellious, nasty, daring, and what's the word? Sexy.

Some of the heaviest hitters from all over the world were assembled. A Romanian doctor named Natasha was there with her slave. She reminded me of Morticia from the Addams family. Her black hair hung down her shoulders while her charcoal-dark eyes coolly surveyed the room. She was dressed in a glittery black cat suit with thigh-high boots. In her hands was a leash attached to a man in his fifties, dressed as a pony, with a saddle on his back and a bit in his mouth. Brunhilda—remember her, the 300-pound sidekick who had wrapped her slave in Saran wrap out by the palm trees?—decided she was ripe for a ride. Hefting her butt cheeks upwards, she hoisted herself aboard the saddle. But no sooner had she taken her seat than the pony rebelled, rearing his head and bucking his back so she fell splat on the floor. I suppressed a giggle. Way to go, ponyboy! Nearby a French woman in a matching horsey outfit, complete with shiny spotted latex hood and horse ears, whinnied and clapped her hooves in triumph.

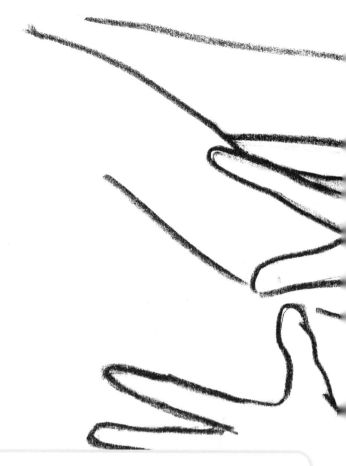

VACATION SEX . . . AT HOME!

For me, vacation sex is best in an exotic locale. However, if you can break free of your familiar constraints by doing it in your kitchen or den, more power to you. Basically it works in any location where you are free to experiment with practices you might not try in your daily routine. If you can manage to clear the papers off the desk, there's no reason you can't take your hedonism into the study (after the kids are safely tucked in bed, of course). But remember, wherever you choose to do it, vacation sex is play sex, free of judgments, free of ordinary moral restrictions—as breezy and carefree as ordering another piña colada.

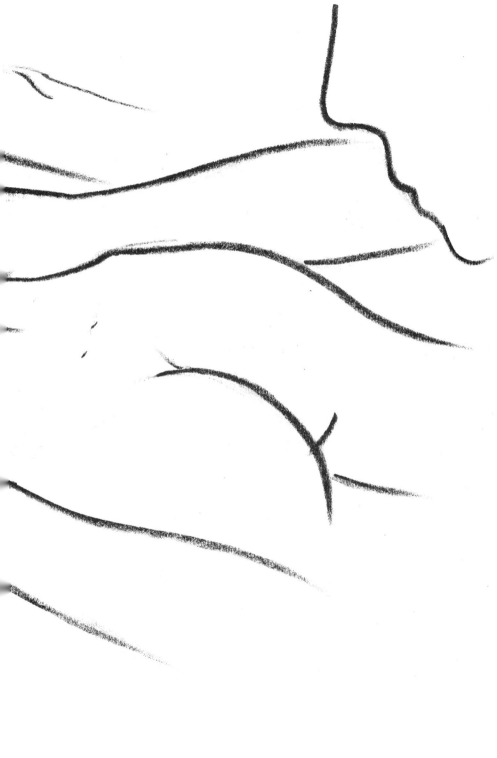

I looked across the room to see what Mistress Siren and her gal pal Pussygalore were up to. Mistress Siren was a petite little number with topaz eyes set in a stunning face of creamy white skin. Pussygalore had bleached her hair almost white. Both were known to be the most vicious of the super-vicious LA contingent that had come in on a private chartered jet. They had strung a naked fifty-year-old man up to the ceiling, and while he was hanging there helpless, they were piercing his cock and balls with needles. The man winced in pain but he obviously reveled in the experience—a true pain slut.

But wait—was that oinking I heard? How could that be? Stepping inside another cool, white room, I spied twelve submissive men and women, all on their knees on the thick rug wearing little masks on their noses—chicken beaks, dog muzzles, and, yes, piggy snouts. Mistress Antoinette was overseeing the bunch. Under her black leather military cap, she had pulled her hair back in a severe ponytail with a very long hairpiece attached, which hung down her backside in a mass of curls. She slapped a black riding crop in her left hand as she marched to and fro perusing her troops. She viciously ordered them to start barking like dogs. Then she had them oink like pigs again.

The velocity of the evening was picking up. I looked back to see how far Mistress Siren and Pussygalore had gotten with their victim. They were doing what's called a "zipper" on his chest—a row of clothespins connected with string. After lovingly attaching them, they told the man to close his eyes and take a deep breath. Then, like a chest wax, they ripped off the zipper hard and fast. His howl was like something out of *The Godfather.*

Just as I thought it couldn't get any wilder, I heard a trumpet call from the beach to signal the start of the kinky wedding. A couple from Colorado had decided they wanted to renew their vows. A bunch of us from the dungeon went traipsing out to find a gazebo that had been festooned with tiny candles for the event. The master of ceremonies had already arrived wearing very tight black leather pants, a white ruffled shirt, and a black satin cape lined with purple satin. The air was full of energy and laughter. Two dancing girls in tinkling gold chains and red chiffon harem pants glided in, throwing rose petals. Then followed the happy couple: the bride wearing nothing but a white corset, a white thong, and white patent leather boots so that her ample derriere was proudly exposed. In her hand, she tightly gripped a leash attached to a silver studded collar around her husband's throat. He was about six-foot-two with glasses—someone I would have taken for a computer geek in any other context.

When the vows were exchanged, the dancing girls started twirling with fired-up torches. A wild Bohemian rhapsody was playing in the background while everything seemed to come to a crazy crescendo. At its peak who should show up but Dita Von Teese in a stunning black leather corset with garters, vintage stockings, and a marvelous pair of peep-toe platforms. Grabbing the emcee's whip, she swirled it over her head and cracked it with a deafening snap. Now that was how to end a wedding.

Needless to say, I slept in the next morning.

Torture to Go

Have toys, will travel. You may want to set up some sort of container that will make your sex life portable. It can be as little as a pouch or as large as a trunk, depending on how much you want to bring with you.

What I use is a pleasure satchel—a simple black nylon bag I picked up at Kmart for a few dollars that is easy to fold up when I am traveling. Deciding what to fill it with is one of my greatest pleasures. (Remember the anticipation factor!)

Your fetish boots are a good place
to stuff cosmetics and sex toys; they'll keep
everything from breaking.

First I survey my toys, or torture instruments, if you will. I try to think of what will make a well-rounded play bag and cover all the disciplines. I usually bring a red silk flogger to warm up the skin, as well as a pair of thumb cuffs—which are basically handcuffs for thumbs that secure the wrists together in a unique way. They are small and easy to carry. Often I take a purple deerskin flogger that packs quite a wallop, a lovely purple and black singletail whip, several yards of purple rope for bondage, and a leopard paddle for spanking. A leopard should never be far from her leopard paddle, I always say.

When I'm feeling particularly wicked, I may pack my evil stick—a twelve-inch, two-pronged metal stick attached to a woven leather handle. The handle is black, silver, and red leather. When I pull the two metal sticks back, they deliver a stinging pain to the skin that is guaranteed to make anybody scream. I paid twelve dollars for that little baby, and it was the best twelve bucks I ever spent. What I particularly adore about it is how little effort is involved on my part, and how much wallop it delivers. Imagine slapping that little stick on someone's balls? *Ouch* and *yummmmmm!*

Next I decide on my wardrobe. If you own any particular piece of clothing that your partner adores, definitely include that. It's also fun to buy something new to surprise him or her. Skimpy is key, and sometimes, slutty can be beyond sexy, particularly if you don't usually dress in that manner. (Remember, vacation time is when you can do whatever you want and be whomever you want!)

The last things to go into my bag of goodies are my jewelry and makeup. The makeup has to be intense and dramatic. Try something you don't usually wear, such as a dark red lipstick with lots of gloss. Or sometimes a deep matte crimson from MAC works well. Don't forget to have your manicure and pedicure done in OPI's "I'm Not a Waitress" red.

GET YOUR WIG ON

If you can let go of your ego and accept that your partner loves the idea of getting it on with a mysterious new woman, wigs can be a wonderful toy for the bedroom and on vacation. (Remember Winston's line? "Anyone as beautiful as you must be married.") I have a fake hairpiece that I often bring along—a classic dominatrix long auburn ponytail that I attach to my hair. I also have a white pageboy that is stunning against black latex. Pro Dommes tend to use a clever array of wigs and hairpieces. Give it a whirl.

VACATION SEX PACKING LIST

Rubber flip flops

Sunscreen

Aloe vera gel

Condoms

Lubricant

Flogger

Plastic wrap

Whip

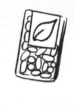
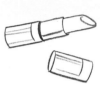
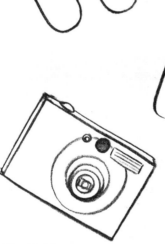
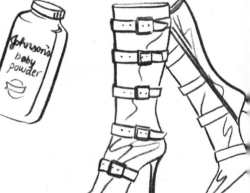

Blindfolds

Costumes

Corset

Wigs

Medical scissors

Needle and thread

Camera

Bottled water

Dildo(s)

Rope

Nipple clamps

Paddles

Vibrator(s)

Fishnets

Pantyhose

Fetish shoes

Fetish boots

Latex clothes

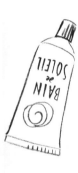

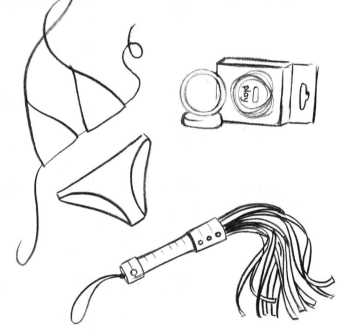

Breath mints

Baby powder

Red lipstick

Red nail polish

Bathing suit
(Think there'll be time
to hit the beach?)

TAKING IT ON THE ROAD
Frequently Asked Questions about Vacation Sex

Is it okay to vacation alone?

Going alone can be difficult because of the loneliness factor. Most of the locals seem to be paired up, and if you're without a partner, management may make you share a less than primo bedroom. On the other hand, being single can be good for threesomes: there seem to be a lot of bisexual women out there. It depends on your head. If you're good at putting yourself out there, it can be interesting because you meet a lot of international people. Generally, though, it's easier to go with a partner or an organized group.

How do I find these groups?

The Internet is your friend. Visit chat rooms, blogs, or websites for kinksters or dominatrixes. Ask your travel agent. Go to "munches" (get-togethers at coffee shops organized by kinky people or groups) or fetish events where a booth or table may be advertising.

Where are the best places to go?

Warm climates seem to bring out the beast. South America is good. Jamaica is great, with three Hedonism resorts (very kinky, mon). Florida has some, too, and throughout the United States there are leather retreats focused on offering the ultimate in S&M play.

What can you do at these places?

Basically anything goes: nude or prude, group sex, bi, lesbian, collars, lace, sex games. Sex happens. Kink events and weekends offer such events as pony play, slave auctions, kinky performers, play parties after hours in official dungeons with monitors, fetish fashion shows, and classes in bondage, whipping, spanking, and electrical play. I once went on a kinky catamaran ride in which a slave was tied to ropes hanging over the water. Slave boys were tied to the mast for whipping, and another slave had an electric vibrator inside him to be turned on whenever his Mistress desired. This can be a bit rough if you are prone to seasickness.

Is there etiquette I should know about?

Most definitely. If you are swinging you always want to ask someone if he or she is interested—never assume that sex with you is something a person wants. Make sure your hygiene is meticulous. Never touch someone else's slave unless you ask if it is okay. Don't crowd a woman if you are a man, couple, or several men. She needs to feel safe. And always, always, have condoms.

Are there obligations?

Enjoy yourself (read: clothes, cell phones, rocks—off).

What are no-nos?

Don't come in the pool.

Any others?

Remember the heat down there. If wrapping someone in cellophane around a palm tree, make sure he's hydrated. And always . . .

Yes?

Try to do it in the shade.

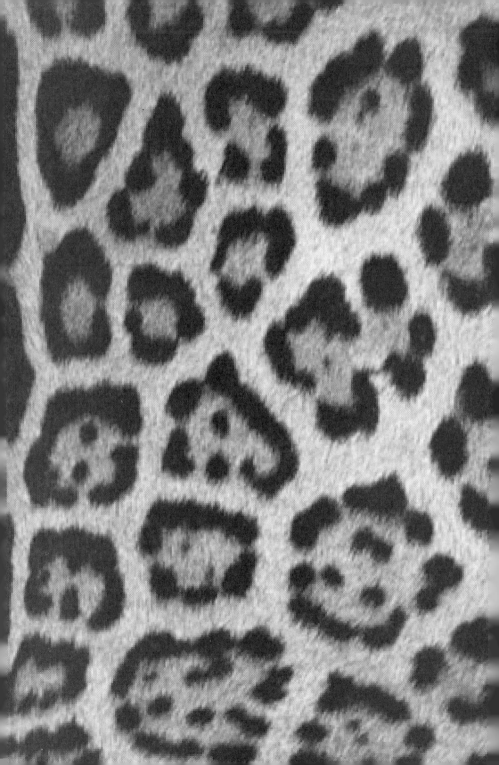

Dungeon
Sale

All good things, they say, must come to an end. And so it was with my time as a professional Domme.

I am an adventurer. I had delved into this world because it brought out all the mischief deep inside me. Along the way it broadened my understanding of the human psyche and somewhat fattened my pocketbook. But it was not doing enough for the side of me that needed attending to. There was so much more to life that interested me—writing, yoga, my spiritual life. I enrolled in classes to study the tomes of Carl Jung, Teilhard de Chardin, and the mystics. I started conversing with a Franciscan brother once a month to seek out what more there is to the human plight than just existing on this planet. I started to have a deeper understanding of how to live in coordination with a higher power that is within us and throughout the universe. It enabled me to connect with and understand what my fellow human beings might be going through. As a result, I felt a new inner peace and joy when I woke up in the morning and faced my day.

You know what I most wanted after all was said and done? After all the experiences I had gone through, all the fireworks, all the hilarity, and all the passion? It came down to this: I wanted a man in my life for an intimate, supportive, and loving relationship unlike anything I had ever experienced before. Believe it or not—and you probably will believe it if you've been reading between the lines—I'm a big believer in romance. I wanted to be able to go with my sweetie to art shows, enjoy romantic dinners in little ethnic restaurants, make dinner at home on a Sunday night before curling up together to watch a movie and fuck our brains out all over the house. Someone with whom I could have a creatively fun and erotic sex life. We'd still be twisted, sure, but our excursions into kink would be one aspect of our lives, not the totality of our existence.

I decided to pull my Website off the Internet and resume working full-time as a clinical psychotherapist. I had always based my private practice around erotic minorities—people who participated in BDSM and other fetishes. My plan was to become a clinical sexpert and use my experience, combined with my academic training, to support people in the Scene and make sure they had healthy self-images. I also wanted to become a public speaker, educating people as to how this could be a healthy and fun endeavor as opposed to something sick and shameful.

I knew my higher power was on my side when I applied to work at a beautiful clinic a hop, skip, and a jump down the street from me. They even offered insurance—thank God. (Dominatrixes don't have a union that provides insurance, unfortunately.) I acquired a position right away and was absolutely thrilled.

However, I did not write on my résumé that I had been a dominatrix. Most people have a hard enough time grasping the concept of a dominatrix with intelligence, compassion, morals, and a love of God—never mind being a psychotherapist to boot. Nor did I tell men, on a first date, that I had been a pro Domme. That would have been the equivalent of pinning a scarlet *D* to my chest. On dates I tended to wait till we reached a point of greater intimacy before I spilled the beans, and if they understood how much extra heat my background could bring to our sex life, all the better. If they couldn't handle it, it wasn't meant to be. No way was I about to be ashamed over a craft and an art form I had spent years perfecting.

To really set myself free, I decided I needed to break down my dungeon and have a dungeon sale. The idea came from Lady Stinger, who had a dungeon sale when she moved out of state. It seemed like a great idea, and the extra cash could come in handy. The first thing on my list was to sell a good majority of my toys. I still wanted to keep some for my personal use and abuse.

It was amazing how much paraphernalia I had accumulated in two years: dildos, attachable steel fingernails, paddles, riding crops, singletail whips, books of erotica, large rolls of Saran wrap, handcuffs, thumb cuffs, a violet wand, and a hell of a lot of clothespins. The list went on and on. I lined everything up on the floor and tables and ticketed each item with a sales tag. How to put a price tag on this stuff, when each item came loaded with a pang of emotion? I contacted everyone I knew by e-mail. People came and went, and I ended up with a few hundred dollars. The sum hardly seemed commensurate to all the pleasure and pain these toys had witnessed.

Then came the big items, starting with my 850-pound cage, which I sold to an old boyfriend who was in the Scene. He was a six-foot-tall scientist who tested tsetse flies for a living. He showed up with his usual scraggly hair, hippie tie-dyed shirt, and light pink corduroy pants, accompanied by his scientist girlfriend, who was tall, skinny, pale, and scraggly. She obviously felt a bit intimidated around me, especially when he instructed her I wouldn't be lifting a finger to help. "For God's sake, Ingrid, she's a Mistress!" They set about taking the door off the hinges of the apartment so the cage would fit through, then sliding the thing on a huge beach towel so it wouldn't scratch the floor. While they were grunting and sweating, I regaled the girlfriend with ideas for how she could have fun with the cage. For instance, she could tie up Mr. Tsetse inside and watch while he jerked himself off. Or she could stand in the cage herself, and he could fuck her through the rods of the door from behind. He thanked me while his girlfriend scrunched her eyebrows.

When one of my neighbors noticed a cage being moved, they asked about it. "It was for my pet monkey," I replied.

When they finally left, I set about getting rid of the bondage bed. I put an ad on eBay, but they promptly notified me that they couldn't post anything of such an adult nature on their site. Oh, grow up, will you please? So I posted it in their adult section as a massage bed. One glimpse of the photo would tell you it wasn't any massage bed, darlin'! Not with all those leather straps and hooks hanging off it. I also sent letters to Mistresses all over the state and anyone I knew in the Scene inquiring if they wanted to buy it. Apparently there was a surfeit at the moment. What a drag. How in the world could there not be a bigger market for a seven-foot, three-inch bondage bed engineered specifically for cock and ball torture? I finally had to give it away to a Mistress with a pickup truck.

In the meantime, one of my clients who was a worthy slave, Pony Boy (he specialized in being a pony and liked to be attached to

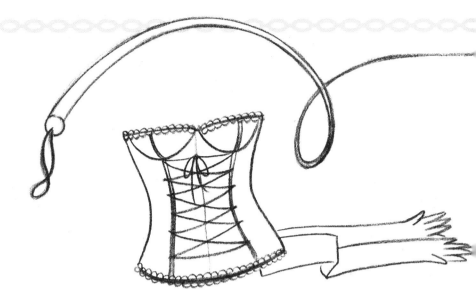

ILONA PARIS ON BEING A PROFESSIONAL DOMINATRIX

As a professional dominatrix, I have learned so much about the human body and what makes it tick. I've seen how the body can absorb pleasure as well as pain and learned the physical effects certain toys can have on the anatomy.

I have also augmented my understanding of human psychology. The mental gymnastics of submission and domination provide a window into the psychological underpinnings that men and women carry with them in their everyday lives. I've seen how the human mind works under stress—both the physical sort and the sort we might classify as the art of the mind fuck. When "playing" with someone, I am choreographing an incredible journey for them. My clients are brought to a wonderful head space and feel high for some time after. It should have the effect of a good therapy session, inducing a feeling of peace and inner strength, free from everyday constraints.

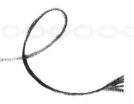

And let's not forget that another delightful benefit of being a dominatrix is that submissives buy you fabulous gifts—boots, perfume, fetishwear, and toys. You have a certain aura as a dominatrix. People are frequently in awe of you, which is a fun thing to experience.

On the other hand, the negative consequences of being a Domme can permeate your life quite deeply. It's exhausting, both physically and psychologically. It can be dangerous working so intimately with people who are, at least at first, essentially strangers. And it's difficult to have a healthy love life outside the dungeon. It takes a very well-grounded, secure man to enter into a relationship with a Domme without feeling outgunned, as it were.

Life for me is about evolving as a human being, continuing to grow and nurture myself and those I love around me. I have seen too many Dommes lose themselves, forget their humanity, and become the bitches they portray. It's not worth the challenge if that's going to happen.

Choosing this as a career is equivalent to being a tightrope walker. It is highly exhilarating—but the chances of falling off that rope and losing your sense of self and enlightenment are very dangerous.

Of course, choosing to be dominant in the privacy of your bedroom with someone you know very well . . . hey, nothing wrong with that.

a cart while carrying about a Mistress) called and asked if he could be of assistance to me in some way.

"Well, slut, funny you should ask . . . "

Ask and ye shall receive. I made arrangements for everyone to come over the next Saturday morning to haul the bed away. As the day approached, my anxiety level skyrocketed. There was a lot attached to this part of my life. I was closing the door on it. It felt good, but there was a small part of me that didn't want to give it up.

Of course, on Saturday everything went wrong that could go wrong. The pickup truck broke down on the way. The bondage bed seemed to be put together with all sorts of hidden glue, nuts, and bolts. Pony Boy, who was acting more like a pack mule helping me dismantle it, went out to buy an array of small saws. It was lunchtime when all of this came to a head; I couldn't wait to explain to my neighbors what this monstrosity was doing coming out of my apartment in bits and pieces. My anxiety level was reaching heights I never thought possible. Finally I did what every good Mistress would do. Putting my slave in charge of the situation, I downed a Haldol and met my girlfriend for lunch. I must say it was a very pleasant lunch: fettuccine with clam sauce, as I recall. When I came home the only sign of my big, beautiful bondage bed was a little scratch on the floor. I sat down in my purple tufted clamshell of a chair, gave my cat Sushi a pat, and let out a deep sigh. It was certainly the end of an era for me.

But just because I had graduated to another place didn't mean I couldn't enjoy the fruits of my experience! I wanted to evolve to a new place where I could educate people about the benefits and joys of this lifestyle. That's why I've included a glorious assortment of tips (see "The Nitty Gritty") to help you to prepare a session, from filling your closet with latex and assembling a toy chest, to setting up your own dungeon in the privacy of your home—complete with a few cautions. Because this is life you're playing with here, darlings. Your own and someone else's. Treat it with respect.

Remember always, in the words of the poet, philosopher and scholar John O'Donohue:

The human person is a threshold where many infinities meet.
The infinity that haunts everyone and which no one can finally quell
is the infinity of one's own interiority.
It is where the private, inner world of a person protrudes into the
anonymous world.
There is a secret relationship between our physical being and the
rhythm of our soul.
The body is the place where the soul shows itself.

And in the immortal words of Ilona Paris:

Be free of the chains that bind you—unless you strap them on
for fun!

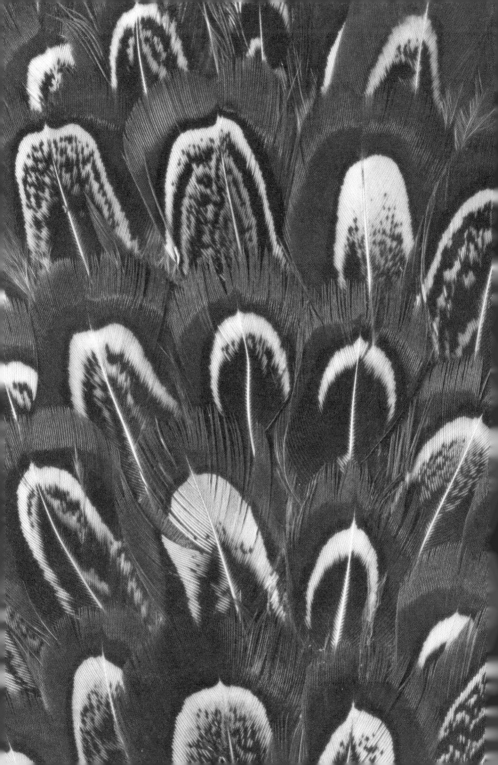

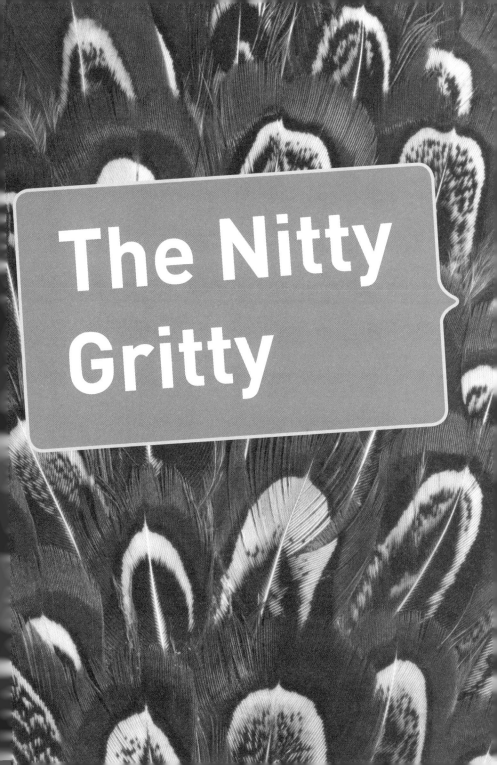

The Nitty Gritty

SETTING UP SHOP

Out with the old and in with the new! Toss out that old pool table and put in a bondage bed! Get rid of the seventies bar and put in a sex hammock!

But first things first. Start small by dedicating one private chest of drawers or one closet to place or hang your favorite sex toys. Put a lock on it so prying eyes can't get in, and call it your toy chest. The Sears Craftsman chest, which I favor, comes with a lock and key. Toss in all the things that turn you on most. I prefer to have each drawer dedicated to a particular theme. One is for vintage stockings, another is for collars and cuffs, and another is for my Hitachi vibrators. I have one drawer for miscellaneous small things, such as tiny vibrators, knives, batteries, Band-aids, breath mints, baby clothespins, and giant black shoelaces.

Here's what I did when I set up my professional dungeon. (You don't have to go this far, obviously, to enjoy sexual mischief with a partner of your own choosing.)

In a specially equipped room in my upscale condo, my dungeon was truly fit for a queen. First, I painted the walls a smashing shade of forest green and installed a throne that had belonged to a wonderful Domme, a burgundy velvet Queen Victoria number. It had karma written all over it. A massive leather whipping wall was covered with hooks to attach handcuffs and ropes. A giant bondage bed was equipped with a pulley so my tied-up and upside-down victims could be lifted into the air for sensory deprivation. Golden locks secured an 850-pound cage that was truly a beautiful thing. It was the size of a telephone booth and made out of real jail-cell bars painted black. It had a door with a lock attached. You could stand it up or lie it down. I felt it was more comfortable standing up. My favorite thing to do with it was tie a man up inside it spread-eagled. Of course, I blindfolded him and then did all kinds of evil things to him once he was made helpless. I had a leopard and leather spanking bench made for me by one of the best fetish-furniture craftsmen out in LA. I also had a portable toilet seat. You never know.

I went to a mountain-climbing store and bought a harness to hang people inside my cage. You should have seen the look on the salesclerk's face when I said, "I want a harness to hang someone inside a cage. Do you have something like that?" It's always nice to shock the help. I have to say I rather enjoyed that little shopping escapade.

I recommend that you go to your local Pier One or Crate and Barrel. Buy unique baskets to hold rope and other accoutrements. Umbrella stands or big vases can make interesting containers for such things as riding crops, paddles, and canes.

Ideas for Your Bed

How you set up your bed depends on what sort of play you are planning to engage in. Messy or clean? Food or bondage? If it is for bondage you will need to decide what type of rope you want to use. I recommend hemp or nylon. Hemp holds nicely. It isn't slippery. It's natural feeling and seems to work better with the skin. Nylon can burn and is a bit more difficult to knot. On the other hand, it is slippery, which is a sensual bonus. You should have both ropes in various lengths of 25, 50, and 100 feet, depending on whether you want to perform an elaborate hog-tie or just want to secure

TOY BOX

Band-aids	Medical scissors
Batteries	Medical tape
Duct tape	Breath mints
Stockings	Cuffs
Leashes	Leather hood
Latex hood	Nylon hood
Pilot earmuffs	Earplugs
Blindfolds	Clothespins (various sizes)
Plastic wrap	Giant black shoestrings
Rope	Leather mitts
Mountain-climbing clips	Handcuffs
Thumb cuffs	Elastic bands
Ball gag	Vibrators
Electric toothbrush	BenGay
Stinging wand	Metal fingernails
Wooden hairbrush	Lingerie
Metal locks	Cock rings
Candles	Lubricant
Nipple clamps	Violet wand
Butt plugs	Kama Sutra Oil of Love
Asian suction cups	Condoms
Capsaicin cream	

someone's wrists. Big, fat electrical duct tape in red or black is fun to use, too. Keep a pair of medical scissors nearby. Have a towel in case you need to place it between knees or ankles that might rub together. Check the bed to make sure it is sturdy wherever you are tying rope to it.

If you are going to be messy, you have a few options. Use medical pads that can be placed under your bottom to catch the juice, so to speak. You can use towels or rubber sheets or even an old plastic shower curtain. If you are in a fix and need something in a hurry, try an unused garbage bag.

Stuff for Your Craftsman Pleasure Chest

Buying toys at conventions was a hoot for me: I bought whips, floggers, butt plugs, lube, flavored condoms, and rubber gloves. But my best purchase—an electric toothbrush—came from CVS. I used the toothbrush on the tip of the cock. Drove men wild. So next time you see a sultry woman in the toothbrush aisle of CVS, check her out. You never know. I have shopped anywhere and everywhere.

An electric golf ball cleaner will also do the trick. No puns intended.

WARDROBE

I also got myself a wardrobe, and here's where even a do-it-yourselfer can go wild. The shoes alone! My faves were my trademark leopard sandals, which I ordered in silver, cobalt-blue, and six other colors. Another pair featured an acrylic upper so foot worshippers could observe all the muscles and veins in my feet during a session. When I put on my red latex gown for the first time, it seemed to confer magical powers on me. I felt like clicking my six-inch patent leather fetish heels and saying, "There's no place like my dungeon."

The fetish clothes I purchased really created a sense of the powerful domina I wanted to portray to the world: rubber latex dresses, black gowns with slits all the way up my thigh, red Mistress zip-tit dresses. Bet you can't guess where the zippers were. It was kind of like wearing a giant elastic, but darling, it looked marvelous!

Soundproofing Your Dungeon

Neighbors tend to get a bit nervous when they hear screaming, groans, and people pleading, "Please don't hurt me." It is wise to use padding to soundproof your dungeon area. Use a thick rug on the floor with padding underneath. I hung beautiful tapestries on my walls. You can also use cork tiles on the floor and walls, which look pretty cool when they are black.

Lighting and Interior Design

The standard colors for dungeons are usually black and purple, but be creative. I used a forest green on my walls with tapestries, gold mirrors, and deep-red velvet and leopard furniture. Make it sumptuous and sexy. Use candles, but keep an eye on them. When things get rough, they can tip over. Bright lights are unforgiving on nude bodies. Use a variety of lighting options to soften the mood and make it mysterious.

Music

Get a good sound system. Music can be a stimulating or soothing accompaniment to your scenes. It can inspire your movements with a whip, or help settle everything down after a rousing session. I use anything from classical to Grace Jones to a global beat. Vendors sell music just for this purpose at some of the fetish fairs.

WHERE TO BUY

Clothing

The Baroness
530B East 13th Street
New York, NY 10009
212-529-5964
www.baroness.com

Delicious Corsets
1040 North American Street #901
Philadelphia, PA 19123
215-413-0375
www.deliciouscorsets.com

Demask
144 Orchard Street
New York, NY 10002
212-466-0814
www.demask.com

Stormy Leather
1158 Howard Street
San Francisco, CA 94103
415-626-1672
www.stormyleather.com

Whiplash
7864 Gloria Avenue
Van Nuys, CA 91406
818-376-7588
www.whiplashusa.com

Purple Passion
211 West 20th Street
New York, NY 10011
212-807-0486
www.purplepassion.com

Syren
7225 Beverly Boulevard
Los Angeles, CA 90036
323-936-6693
www.syren.com

Tony Shoes
6505 Hollywood Boulevard
Hollywood, CA 90028
323-467-5604
www.tonyshoesinc.com

Leather Man
111 Christopher Street
New York, NY 10014
212-243-5339
www.theleatherman.com

Agent Provocateur
133 Mercer Street
New York, NY 10012
212-965-0229
www.agentprovocateur.com

O.K. Uniform
368 Broadway
New York, NY 10013
212-791-9789
www.okuniform.com

Toys

- Sex shops
- The Internet
- eBay
- Fetish events or fairs
- Medical stores
- Hardware stores
- Home Depot
- Drugstores
- Grocery stores
- Garden shops

Check with friends when buying toys. The basic rule is to buy what you like and what turns you on. If a friend has something that catches your eye, ask her where she got it. Check through blogs or chat rooms to find out where people are getting things. Join a society or group and ask people what they suggest. Be creative and try anything. Once you open your mind, you will find that you can buy toys anywhere: the hair-care section in a store; the utensil department in Crate and Barrel; the rope and chain section in Home Depot. Anything goes, my friends.

MedicalToys.com
3144 Broadway, Suite #4-245
Eureka, CA 95501-3838
800-791-3931
www.MedicalToys.com

Condomania
351 Bleecker Street
New York, NY 10014
212-691-9442
www.condomania.com

Eve's Garden
119 W. 57th Street Suite 1201
New York, NY 10019
800-848-3837
www.evesgarden.com

Toys in Babeland
43 Mercer Street
New York, NY 10013
212-966-2120
www.babeland.com
4 locations, see Website

Eros Boutique
581A Tremont Street
Boston, MA 02118
617-425-0345
www.erosboutique.com

Hubba Hubba
534 Massachusetts Avenue
Cambridge, MA 02139
617-492-9082

QUESTIONS TO ASK YOUR PLAYING PARTNER PRIOR TO A SCENE

Okay, so you've decided you want to play—but you still need to make sure you check in with your play partner before you begin. These are the questions to ask.

- Do you have any medical issues I need to know about such as arthritis, bad joints, recent or old surgery?
- Have you had any dental work done recently?
- Are you wearing contact lenses?
- Are you having your period?
- Is your asshole clean?
- Are there any issues with your urethra?
- Have you taken any drugs or alcohol prior to this session?
- Do you have any phobias or fears I need to know about?
- Do you have any issues with abuse?
- Do you have any spinal issues?

Decide on a Safe Word

The safe word is a verbal cue the submissive (or bottom) gives to the dominant (or top) to alert him or her to slow down or stop. You can use classic words such as "green" or "red," or come up with something that works for you. You are not playing safe if you do not agree on this, and don't let anyone tell you otherwise.

Warnings

I would be remiss if I did not remind you, as you embark on adventures of your own, that as someone who will take another's body and psyche in your hands, you are entrusted with a special responsibility not to fuck it up.

Be intuitive and hypersensitive to the wonderful human being before you.

You have to do all this from a state of mental stability.

You never want to take out your frustrations or your anger on your partner.

And again, I can't stress this enough: **Always be safe, sane, and consensual.**

SO YOU WANT TO BE A DOMINATRIX?

How does one go about getting training to become a Mistress?

You need to take classes just as if you were going to school. I cannot express the importance of learning as much as you can. A whip is a very dangerous thing and takes a lot of practice. You need many classes in bondage, candles, fireplay, safety, asphyxiation, caning, paddling, vampirism, fisting, the anatomy of the penis and vagina, knifeplay, and so on.

One should never go hunting without experience, and never without guidance. The same goes with any relationship, especially S&M. A person wouldn't buy a house without doing research, would she? Hopefully, a person would not get married without knowing plenty about his partner. The same things are true for people who practice S&M.

Where do I start?

Find fetish events or societies that feature training classes. Once again, look on the Internet. Dominatrix sites frequently have Website links that can be full of information. Try blogs and chat rooms.

Fetish or sex shops sometimes have listings. Pump the sales help for advice. Fetish books may also offer listings in the back of the book, which can be quite helpful.

There are many ways you can start to become familiar with the Scene. You may choose to go to a club that features BDSM play. These clubs can be found in magazines for dominatrixes.

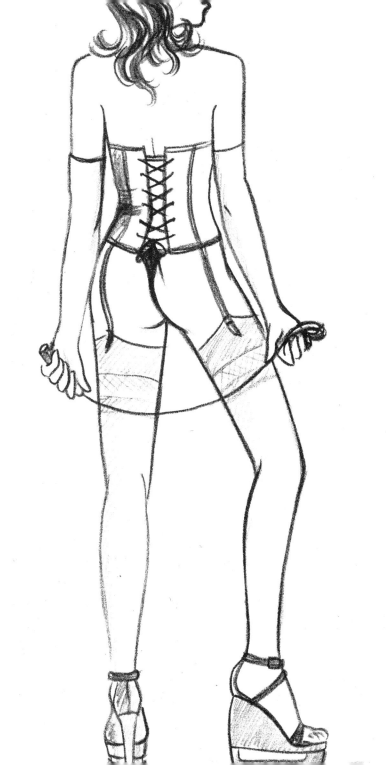

The backs of kink magazines, such as *Skin Two*, have a plethora of listings for you to explore. If there is a fetish event in your community, organizations such as the Boston Dungeon Society will have tables featuring paraphernalia and discussions of their offerings. Sometimes bulletin boards in clubs or sex shops may feature flyers. There are books on the lifestyle such as *Screw the Roses, Send Me the Thorns: The Romance and Sexual Sorcery of Sadomasochism* by Philip Miller and Molly Devon. This book has a wonderful reference section at the end. Frequently books will have listings in the back according to state or country. Or you may want to join a private community such as a leather club. The club will feature lectures on such topics as spanking, caning, finding a Dom(me), vampire play, spirituality in S&M, and so on. They also sponsor get-togethers called "munches" where people meet in coffee shops with other like-minded kinksters.

Fetish events are another resource. We have the Fetish Flea Market in Boston, but I have been to events all over the world. These events feature dinners, parties, and vendors that sell toys and equipment. They also feature lectures, which can be very helpful in your training. These are usually advertised in alternative newspapers in the alternative lifestyle or sex sections of a bookstore.

The most widely available resource to meet people is the Internet. Try sites such as AdultFriendFinder.com and Alt.com. Craig's List has a kink chat room (Craigslist.org). The well-known author Dr. Gloria G. Brame has a wonderful Website full of information for kinksters (Gloria-Brame.com). Look for blogs on kink. Sites for dominatrixes are rich with information and chat rooms.

List a vanilla personal ad, but put in a few words that a kinkster would pick up on such as "dominant," "like to serve my partner," "like to clean a lot," "I am into feet," "I am into alternative lifestyles," "I enjoy leather and lingerie," or "women should be worshipped."

Find a sub and practice, practice, practice. *Heeheeheeheehee*.

Where do I get training for safety?

Try the Red Cross or the American Heart Association in your city. If in doubt, ask your doctor or call a hospital. You need to know how to resuscitate someone or treat a person who has been hurt until you can get professional help. When in doubt, call 911 for an ambulance immediately. Make the call first and then apply first-aid.

What do I do about safety for myself?

Working in a dungeon with other women helps with the security level. If you work alone, as most Dommes do, make sure you do a thorough phone interview. Call other Dommes the client has seen for references. Make a safe call. This means you call a trusted person to give him or her the client's name and phone number prior to the session, and call again after the session to let the person know you are all right. If you have enough money, you can hire a security guard, or you may be lucky enough to have a slave do it for free. If you are alone with a new client, tie him down right away.

Again, communication is all-important. One of the most distinguishing characteristics of a BDSM relationship is the openness, the continuous communication that occurs. This is vitally important, because the guide words are safe, sane, and consensual.

Do I need a lawyer?

The first thing I did was get a lawyer. I wanted to make sure I was protected and wasn't going to be thrown in the stocks for a public stoning. Laws pertaining to S&M vary from state to state, and you need to make sure that your lawyer is kink-friendly and able to advocate aggressively on your behalf. I found mine through my local leather society.

What questions should I ask a prospective client who wants to set up an appointment?

Ask the person's name, age, phone number, and height and weight. Is he married or in a relationship so you need to be careful of marking? Has he played before, for how long, and with whom? Don't be afraid to call that person. What does he like to see a dominatrix wear? Does he have any physical problems you should know about? What are his favorite fetishes or fantasies?

FINAL THOUGHTS

Well folks, it's been great. I took it easy on you in this book to break you in gently. So stay tuned for my next set of adventures, which promises to be chock full of more deviousness and fun.

In the meantime, may you continue to grow stronger in your pursuits.

As for me, I enjoy life more now than ever. I am grateful that my head is in a good place, and that my spiritual strength is expanding. Sitting as I do on the board of the National Leather Association's Domestic Violence Project with a few other psychological heavyweights, I think of myself as an advisor to the community, someone with enough wisdom and practical insight to act as a guide. Just last night I counseled a new client, seated on the velvet throne that I now use as a rather regal office chair. As a member of an "erotic minority," her plight was classic for someone who had sought help in the vanilla world of treatment. She spoke with great hurt about how her previous counselor used to grow quiet with disapproval whenever she spoke of her sexual proclivities. As I listened, I acknowledged to myself how often I had heard that same story. The poor counselor was just too nervous and uptight—too limited in her experience in the real world of sex—to be of any help to anyone in this arena.

I am so happy and excited to be the counselor I am today, someone who believes it is okay to be luscious, juicy, kinky, creative and do what you want to do sexually. I like the fact that I practice what I preach. I see the smiles on my clients' faces when I share my past with them. It is so exciting to me to be a beacon in the sky, lighting a path to sexual freedom. When I go into a counseling session these days, I feel as if I am flying. The people I work with are intelligent, fun, and focused. They are so appreciative to speak with a sexpert who finally understands them.

Oh, I admit I still pout a little bit every now and then that that part of my life is over. I still get a little twinge of sadness when I come across an item stuck here and there in a closet or behind a door: a roll of Saran wrap, or a dildo shaped like Bill Clinton. I kept all my fetish shoes and clothes, and sometimes I go into the back of my closet and trail my hands over the latex or put on my platform boots and strut around my apartment. They tug at my heart, these little things that will always remind me of my unusual pathway through life—one that helped me gain control, made up for all the bad that ever happened to me, and gave me a sense of mastery in my life. Being a dominatrix was such a cool thing to do, and I always loved a good laugh. But mostly I'm delighted to be where I am. Besides, I may just blow everyone's mind and show up in full regalia again someday. Or maybe I'll have them bury me in my bright red latex Mistress dress. Wouldn't that be a hoot!?

> *May you be able to journey to that place in your soul*
>> *where there is great love, warmth, feeling, and forgiveness.*
> *May this change you.*
> *May you be brought into the real passion, kinship, and*
>> *affinity of belonging.* —**John O'Donohue**

And so, dear reader, the light in me salutes the light in you. *Namaste.*

The Paris Report
Methodology

This survey was created specifically to research the characteristics of practitioners of sadomasochism. The first page contained eleven fill-ins that pertained to gender (male or female), age, race, religion, and sexual orientation (heterosexual, bisexual, gay and other). The level of education was of interest along with the income factor. Did participants use mood enhancers such as alcohol, marijuana, opiates, or other substances and how often? It has been hypothesized that people who participate in sadomasochism have abuse in their backgrounds, so participants were asked if they had ever experienced sexual abuse or domestic violence in their lives. Respondents were asked at what age they had experienced their first kinky thought and their first kinky activity, with opportunity to describe. The last open-ended question asked people at what age did they feel they became a member of the S&M community, with the opportunity to describe the event or life experience.

The survey was distributed at the Fetish Flea Market in Boston in December 2004 to a non-random sample. The respondents were 120 women, 154 men, 6 transgenders, and 24 respondents who did not identify their sex. I compiled statistical data with the help of a statistician.

Bibliography

Andrews, Grant. *The 43rd Mistress: A Sensual Odyssey*. California: Greenery Press, 2000.

Apostolides, Marianne. "The Pleasure of Pain," *Psychology Today*, September/October 1999.

Arsan, Emmanuelle. *Emmanuelle*. New York: Grove Press, 1971.

Bentley, Toni. *The Surrender: An Erotic Memoir*. New York: Regan Books, 2004.

Brame, Gloria G., *Domina: The Sextopians*. Florida: Universal Publishers, 1998.

Brame, Gloria G., William D. Brame, and Jon Jacobs. *Different Loving: The World of Dominance and Submission*. New York: Villard, 1993.

Brothers, Joyce. *Boston Globe Sunday Magazine*, February 27, 2005.

Burton, Sir Richard, and F. F. Arbuthnot. *The Pop-Up Kama Sutra*. New York: Stewart, Tabori and Chang, 2003.

Cowan, Lyn. *Masochism: A Jungian View*. Connecticut: Spring Publications, Inc., 1982.

"The Fantasy Issue," *Glamour Magazine*, April 2007.

Hollander, Xaviera. *The Happy Hooker: My Own Story*. New York: Dell Publishing Group, 1972.

Janus, Samuel S., PhD, and Cynthia L. Janus, MD. *The Janus Report on Sexual Behavior*. New York: John Wiley and Sons, Inc., 1993.

Jong, Erica. *Parachutes and Kisses*. London: Panther Books, 1984.

Kinsey, Alfred, Wardell Pomeroy, Clyde Martin, and Paul Gebhard. *Sexual Behavior in the Human Female*. Philadelphia and London: W. B. Saunders Co., 1953.

Kleinplatz, Peggy J., and Charles Moser, eds. *Sadomasochism: Powerful Pleasures*. Philadelphia: Harrington Park Press, 1988.

Midori. *The Seductive Art of Japanese Bondage*. California: Greenery Press, 2001.

Miller, Philip and Molly Devon. *Screw the Roses, Send Me the Thorns: The Romance and Sexual Sorcery of Sadomasochism*. Fairfield: Mystic Rose Books, 1988.

Nin, Anaïs. *Delta of Venus: Erotica*. New York and London: Harcourt Brace Jovanovich, 1969.

Noyes, John K. *The Mastery of Submission: Inventions of Masochism*. New York: Cornell University Press, 1997.

Phillips, Anita. *A Defense of Masochism*. New York: St. Martin's Press, 1998.

Reage, Pauline. *The Story of O*. New York: Ballantine Books, 1981.

Reik, Theodor. *Of Love and Lust: On the Psychoanalysis of Romantic and Sexual Emotions*. New York: Jason Aronson, 1974.

Roquelaure, A. N. (Anne Rice). *Beauty's Punishment*. New York: Plume, 1990.

———. *Beauty's Release*. New York: Plume, 1990

———. *The Claiming of Sleeping Beauty*. New York: Plume, 1990.

Sade, Marquis de. Justine, *Philosophy in the Bedroom, and Other Writings*. New York: Grove Press, 1990.

Silverberg, Cory. "Anal Sex Statistics." http://sexuality.about.com:80/od/sexinformation/a/anal_sex_stats.htm.

Bland, Lucy, and Laura Doan. *Sexology Uncensored: The Documents of Sexual Science*. Chicago: University of Chicago Press, 1999.

University of Michigan Health System. "Pleasure and Pain: Study Shows Brain's 'Pleasure Chemical' Is Involved in Response to Pain Too." *Science Daily*, October 19, 2006. http://www.sciencedaily.com/releases/2006/10/061019094148.htm.

Acknowledgments

I would like to thank Timothy Flapp, my co-writer, for his devotion, belief, terrific writing, and debauched sense of thinking. (He might even show a few claw marks from the whole experience.) I am forever grateful to Ann Treistman, my editor, for her fierce pursuit of getting me to write this book, which brought tears to my eyes. And then there is Jennifer Unter, my agent, who serves as a combination counselor and pit bull when needed. These three people form an incredible team who honor me with their support.

I must thank my family for their unconditional love. It ain't easy having a dominatrix and a therapist as an auntie. I must thank my best friend, Mark, who has held my hand, wiped my tears, and reminded me it is all about the cock! Thanks to my friends, the May Babies, and you know who you are darlings. Lastly, thanks to Brother John and my friends and teachers of The Guild for Spiritual Learning.